· AMERICA'S AGING ·

Health in an Older Society

Committee on an Aging Society
Institute of Medicine and National Research Council

NATIONAL ACADEMY PRESS
Washington, D.C. 1985

National Academy Press • 2101 Constitution Avenue, NW • Washington, DC 20418

NOTICE: The project that is the subject of this report was approved by the Governing Board of the National Research Council, whose members are drawn from the councils of the National Academy of Sciences, the National Academy of Engineering, and the Institute of Medicine. The members of the committee responsible for the report were chosen for their special competences and with regard for appropriate balance.

This report has been reviewed by a group other than the authors according to procedures approved by a Report Review Committee consisting of members of the National Academy of Sciences, the National Academy of Engineering, and the Institute of Medicine.

The Institute of Medicine was chartered in 1970 by the National Academy of Sciences to enlist distinguished members of the appropriate professions in the examination of policy matters pertaining to the health of the public. In this, the Institute acts under both the Academy's 1863 congressional charter responsibility to be an adviser to the federal government and its own initiative in identifying issues of medical care, research, and education.

This study has been supported by funds from the National Research Council Fund, a pool of private, discretionary, nonfederal funds that is used to support a program of Academy-initiated studies of national issues in which science and technology figure significantly. The NRC Fund consists of contributions from a consortium of private foundations including the Carnegie Corporation of New York, the Charles E. Culpeper Foundation, the William and Flora Hewlett Foundation, the John D. and Catherine T. MacArthur Foundation, the Andrew W. Mellon Foundation, the Rockefeller Foundation, and the Alfred P. Sloan Foundation; the Academy Industry Program, which seeks annual contributions from companies that are concerned with the health of U.S. science and technology and with public policy issues with technological content; and the National Academy of Sciences and the National Academy of Engineering endowments. The study was also supported by the Charles A. Dana Foundation.

Library of Congress Cataloging in Publication Data

Committee on an Aging Society (U.S.)
  Health in an older society.

  Includes papers from a symposium held July 18–20,
1983 at the National Academy of Sciences.
  Bibliography: p.
  Includes index.
  1. Aged—Care and hygiene—United States—Congresses.
2. Aged—Diseases—United States—Congresses. I. Title.
[DNLM: 1. Aged. 2. Aging. 3. Health Services Research. 4. Socioeconomic
Factors. WT 30 C7345h] RA564.8.C627 1985   362.1'0880565   85-15321

ISBN 0-309-03543-0

Cover photograph courtesy of the American Association of Retired Persons.

Printed in the United States of America   Second Printing, November 1987

COMMITTEE ON AN AGING SOCIETY

This list shows affiliations of members at the time of their service with the committee.

INSTITUTE OF MEDICINE

Preface

Substantial increases in the number and proportion of older persons in the decades ahead portend significant changes in American society. Indeed, demographic projections of rapid population aging have led some observers to characterize the United States as an "aging society."

The ways in which an aging society might be a different society, in other than demographic characteristics, are not entirely clear. But it is evident that the changing age structure of the population will have major implications with respect to:

- the financing, development, organization, and use of health care resources;
- the patterns of families, social relations, social institutions, living arrangements, and physical environments that constitute the contexts in which individuals age;
- the distribution of jobs—and the earnings, status, and satisfaction that they may provide—among older and younger workers, within the context of age discrimination laws, seniority practices, and technological innovation;
- the economic aspects of providing retirement income through various public and private mechanisms;
- the quality of life of the population across the life course including functional status, well-being, legal status, and personal autonomy; and
- an ever-shifting agenda of other public policy issues.

If we are to cope effectively, our understanding of the specific implications of these demographic changes—for older persons, for age relations, and for the institutions of our society—must be enhanced.

The Committee on an Aging Society was organized to identify selected issues that need to be confronted, soon and in the longer term. Recognizing that many organizations and ad hoc groups have been addressing a range of issues associated with older persons themselves, the committee has attempted to emphasize broader societal issues as well. From those issues the Committee on an Aging Society is suggesting topics that warrant systematic investigations fostered by the National Research Council, Institute of Medicine, and other organizations, which in turn will provide a basis for action by social institutions and policy-makers.

As part of its examination of research implications of the changing age structure of the U.S. population, the Committee on an Aging Society convened a symposium on July 18–20, 1983, at the National Academy of Sciences, on the medical, social, and public policy aspects of long-term health care and related services for chronically ill and disabled older persons. The objective was not to propose national policy but to explore areas of research that might contribute usefully to the weighing of national choices.

This volume is the first of a series in which the committee will put forward suggested issues for attention, based on symposia that explored selected topics. Future reports will consider topics such as productive roles in an aging society, the social and built environment, and legal and ethical issues. This report summarizes the committee's recommendations and the discussions on which they were based and presents the papers commissioned for the symposium on the burden of long-term illness and disability.

FREDERICK C. ROBBINS
President
Institute of Medicine

Contents

SUMMARY   1
    Introduction,   1
    Demographic Aspects of the Older Population,   2
    Dependence and Independence,   6
    Medical Aspects and Prospects,   9
    Services and Mismatches,   14
    Conclusions and Recommendations,   20
    Bibliography and References,   25

WAXING OF THE GRAY, WANING OF THE GREEN   28
    David L. Rabin

ACTIVE LIFE EXPECTANCY: SOCIETAL IMPLICATIONS   57
    Sidney Katz, David S. Greer, John C. Beck,
    Laurence G. Branch, and *William D. Spector*

HEALTH, DISEASE, AND CARDIOVASCULAR AGING   73
    Edward G. Lakatta

DEPRESSIVE ILLNESS IN LATE LIFE 105
    Dan Blazer

AGING AND AGE-DEPENDENT DISEASE: COGNITION AND
    DEMENTIA 129
    Robert Katzman

Informal Social Support Systems for the Frail
  Elderly 153
    Barbara Silverstone

Financing Long-term Care for the Elderly:
  Institutions, Incentives, Issues 182
    Anne R. Somers

Index 235

· AMERICA'S AGING ·

Health in an Older Society

Summary

INTRODUCTION

The aging of the society implies tremendous change in the extent and mix of needs for health care and social services in the United States, not only for people in the retirement years. More Americans (the baby-boom generation) are entering the middle years, in which more of the chronic diseases begin to appear, and over the coming decades the proportion of society over 65 is expected nearly to double. Projections by the Bureau of the Census suggest that between the years 1982 and 2030 the U.S. population will have increased from 231,997,000 to 304,300,000; the median age will have increased from 30.6 years to 40.8 years; and the over-65 portion of the population will have increased from 11.6 to 21.1 percent. People will be living longer, in part because of improved care made possible by medical advances. Those who do suffer disabilities but are otherwise healthy will also live longer. And many Americans, living much longer, will be more likely to incur the debility that can come with problems of very old age.

In this complex of issues there are few, if any, more poignant, more complicated, or more important than the burden of chronic illness and disability among older people. The primary bearers of this burden, it must be remembered, are the older persons who suffer from long-term illness and disability, irrespective of the

1

apportionment of the dollar cost of medical care through the society. It should not be assumed that older persons are uniquely subject to chronic illness and disability; in fact, until relatively late in life most Americans are remarkably healthy. But the circumstances of older persons who are disabled command attention, and the number of Americans of an age at which chronic illness is more likely to occur is growing.

This report addresses health issues of two kinds. First it considers the patterns of age and disability in older persons today and likely patterns in the future. It then considers what kinds of services will be required by an aging society. Biomedical research is beginning to show that aging does not necessarily mean disability, which is a function of disease and injury; with medical advances, patterns of disease and disability among older Americans may change considerably. And expectations about chronic disease affect thinking about long-term care, which in turn raises deep-seated policy questions about the relationships of health and welfare systems. Disability is a product of the interaction between the individual and the environment, including the social environment, and therefore cannot be considered by itself (Hahn, 1984). Other reports resulting from the series of issues to be addressed by the Committee on an Aging Society will consider aspects of these interactions such as productive roles for an aging society, the social and built environment, and legal and ethical issues that also impact health.

DEMOGRAPHIC ASPECTS OF THE OLDER POPULATION

A full statistical portrait of the elderly in the United States does not exist. The National Research Council Committee on National Statistics has begun examining needs for statistical information on the aging population, and the National Center for Health Statistics and the Health Care Financing Administration have begun a series of studies of the health status of older Americans. There are indicative pieces of the picture. A recent summary estimate by the National Center for Health Statistics from its National Health Interview Survey (which excludes resident hospital and nursing home patients and others in the institutionalized population) looks at large age groupings in the noninstitutionalized civilian population and shows disabling chronic conditions rising sharply with age in the group aged 45 to 64 and dramatically among persons 65 and older (Table 1).

Published summary national morbidity statistics for the large 65-and-over group should but do not always differentiate between the young old and the persons who have come to be termed the frail elderly. The term *frail elderly* needs to be defined by statistics to enable collection of information and analysis of data by age groups, such as 66 to 76, 76 to 85, and 85 +. National Health Interview Survey data published less routinely show the proportion of noninstitutionalized persons with chronic limitations of function increasing most markedly for the 85-and-over age group (Table 2). There is no directly comparable survey of the institutionalized population. The last National Nursing Home Survey, in 1977, showed a little over 5 percent of the 65-and-over population to be resident patients in nursing homes; in this group both age and gender differences emerged sharply (Table 3).

The problem is the more pressing because long-term care has not been incorporated fully into the nation's social and health programs, it has received broad public attention only episodically, the numbers of people directly affected are growing, and its dimensions are far from satisfactorily understood. Understanding the functional capabilities of older persons and recog-

TABLE 1 Activity Limitation by Chronic Health Problem, Civilian Noninstitutionalized Population, United States, 1981

Age	Population		Limitation in Activity		Limitation in Major Activity[a]		No Activity Limitation	
	1,000s	%	1,000s	%	1,000s	%	1,000s	%
All	225,048	100.0	32,309	14.4	24,552	10.9	192,739	85.6
<17	58,883	100.0	2,216	3.8	1,153	2.0	56,666	96.2
17–44	97,137	100.0	8,151	8.4	5,219	5.4	88,986	91.6
45–64	44,179	100.0	10,574	23.9	8,444	19.1	33,605	76.1
65 +	24,849	100.0	11,368	45.7	9,736	39.2	13,481	54.3

[a]Major activity refers to ability to work, keep house, or engage in school or preschool activities.

SOURCE: U.S. Department of Health and Human Services. 1982. National Center for Health Statistics, Public Health Service. Vital and Health Statistics, Series 10, No. 141. B. Bloom. Current Estimates from the National Health Interview Survey: United States, 1981. Washington, D.C.: U.S. Government Printing Office: DHHS Publication (PHS) 82-1569.

TABLE 2   Dependency of Civilian Noninstitutionalized Population in Activities of Daily Living,[a] United States, 1979

Age	Population 1,000s	%	Activity Limitation 1,000s	%	No Activity Limitation 1,000s	%
18+	153,178	100.0	4,851	3.2	148,327	96.8
18–44	86,378	100.0	676	0.8	85,702	99.2
45–54	22,744	100.0	526	2.3	22,218	97.7
55–64	20,713	100.0	832	4.0	19,881	96.0
65–74	14,929	100.0	1,043	6.9	13,886	93.1
75–84	6,869	100.0	1,101	16.0	5,768	84.0
85+	1,544	100.0	674	43.6	870	56.4

[a]Activities of daily living include bathing, dressing, using toilet room, mobility, continence, and eating.

SOURCE: U.S. Department of Health and Human Services. 1983. National Center for Health Statistics, Public Health Service. B. A. Feller. Americans Needing Help to Function at Home. Advance data from Vital and Health Statistics of the National Center for Health Statistics, No. 92, September 14, 1983.

nizing needs for long-term health care and related services for the expanding older population are crucial to a consideration of resources for care of the chronically ill in all age groups.

These issues have important economic implications as well, as Medicare, Medicaid, Social Security, and related social and health programs with income-transfer effects are reassessed. The large numbers of people to be served and the intrinsic cost of care keep the national medical bill high. Few Americans can afford to be self-insuring for health care. Medicare coverage is incomplete, private supplementary insurance generally is limited and expensive, a comprehensive set of health care coverages is out of reach for most of the growing number of Americans of retirement age, and a mismatch of insurance and social programs and needs has forced many older Americans into poverty and welfare dependency.

As part of its examination of research implications of the changing age structure of the U.S. population, the Committee on an Aging Society convened a symposium on July 18–20, 1983, at the National Academy of Sciences, on the medical, social, and public policy aspects of long-term health care and related services for chronically ill and disabled older persons. The objective was

TABLE 3 Dependency of Nursing Home Resident Patients in Activities of Daily Living,[a] United States, 1977

	Population		Activity Limitation		No Activity Limitation	
	Number	%	Number	%	Number	%
All	1,303,100	100	1,178,600	90.4	124,500	9.6
Male	375,300	100	324,500	86.5	50,800	13.5
Female	927,800	100	854,100	92.1	73,700	7.9
<65	177,100	100	135,600	76.6	41,500	23.4
65–74	211,400	100	181,900	86.0	29,500	14.0
75–84	464,700	100	431,100	92.8	33,600	7.2
85+	449,900	100	430,100	95.6	19,800	4.4

[a]Activities of daily living include bathing, dressing, using toilet room, mobility, continence, and eating.

SOURCE: U.S. Department of Health and Human Services. 1981. National Center for Health Statistics, Public Health Service. Vital and Health Statistics, Series 13, No. 59. Hing, E. Characteristics of Nursing Home Residents, Health Status, and Care Received: National Nursing Home Survey, United States, May–December 1977. Hyattsville, Md.: National Center for Health Statistics; DHHS Publication (PHS) 81-1712.

not to propose national policy but to explore areas of research that might contribute usefully to the weighing of national choices.

Researchers, public administrators, and the health professions have begun to focus intensively on aspects of functional capacity and long-term care; these are protean problems. There is not yet a sense of an agenda for research needed for their assessment.

Stories of hot-plate fires, nursing home horrors, and old people living in poverty are symptomatic of issues not fully faced. Facing these issues requires recognizing the scale of the problem, the changing demography and health status of the population, institutional elements, issues of individual and organizational values and behavior, pertinent economic issues, and specific problems of disease.

Dorothy P. Rice and Jacob J. Feldman, in a paper adapted from their presentation to the 1982 annual meeting of the Institute of Medicine, observed:

As more people live longer, chronic diseases, most commonly conditions of middle and old age, have emerged as major causes of death and disability. There are now many more persons suffering from conditions that are managed or controlled rather than cured. . . . Because these conditions are often of long duration, they create burdens for the individual and for society. . . .

Only a small proportion—5 percent—of the elderly are in nursing homes, but 22 percent of the very old (85 and over) are in nursing homes. . . . As expected, nursing home residents are older and more dependent than the noninstitutional elderly. . . . In general, these elderly residents suffer from multiple chronic conditions and functional impairments. [Rice and Feldman, 1983]

Assessing these problems is not a straightforward matter of looking solely at the numbers. Census projections show the aging of the society generally. Projective epidemiology and projections of the extent and kinds of social and health services that an older population needs have barely begun; moreover, projections vary greatly, depending on assumptions and definitions made for statistical purposes. Government statistical series tend to define conditions variously in accord with specific programs interests and eligibilities. *Disability* often is narrowly defined for legal purposes; so is *long-term care.* How these terms are defined can affect the numbers significantly. In this report these terms are used broadly.

Rice and Feldman comment:

The accuracy of population projections, regardless of their source, may be questioned. . . . The precise numbers are less important than the need to recognize the problems . . . resulting from the aging population in the future. . . .

Our crystal ball becomes much cloudier when we begin to project . . . trends in the prevalence of ill health and infirmity. . . . It is . . . quite possible that . . . there may be an increasing proportion of individuals in quite good health up to the point of death and an increasing proportion with prolonged severe functional limitation, with a decline in the proportion with an only moderate degree of infirmity.

Turning finally to assumptions regarding the future use of health services, we plunge even deeper into the great abyss. . . . The more highly educated tend to live longer, be in better health, but, relative to their health condition, use more medical care than the less educated.

Of even greater consequences than such demographic factors are, of course, changes in our value structure. [Rice and Feldman, 1983]

DEPENDENCE AND INDEPENDENCE

For most acute cases of disease and injury in the United States there is a well-established, if not always adequate, medical armamentarium from which the treatment of choice is drawn or developed, and if the condition is remediable the patient's long-term well-being is assumed. The disease or the injury is the target of therapy. For chronic, disabling, and degenerative conditions, the issues are far more complex. The condition is the target of therapy here, too, but unless the condition clearly is temporary the patient's long-term well-being cannot be assumed, the range of options for care is less obvious, and decisions about care are more likely to be influenced by perceptions of burdens. Even more than the perceived burden of the condition, it may be the perceived burden of care that dominates decisions about care.

Circumstances and style of care can be important determinants of a patient's ability to function with relative independence, leading as full a life as medical condition permits, but there is no consensus on either definition or goals of long-term care. Moreover, the daily concerns of patient, family, friends, health professionals, and support staff, and the various institutional and organizational habits and imperatives of social service agencies, nursing homes, insurers, and government agencies are unlikely to coincide.

The situations differ substantially. The specific requirements for care of an individual who has long suffered and adjusted to one physical handicap such as loss of a limb are not the same as those for care of a patient with a progressive degenerative disease. Chronic mental illness has its special, varied requirements for patient support. A broken hip may require a long convalescence for an older person, but the requirements for care are very different from the needs of a victim of emphysema. At certain stages, victims of stroke and victims of Alzheimer's disease may be similarly helpless and the kinds of care they need may overlap, but their needs also differ considerably.

Among older people debilities usually stem from many causes. Multiple conditions complicate diagnosis and treatment, and care is a yet more elusive concept. The effects of degenerative disease become evident; the requirements for long-term care are complex; and the combination of debility, stress, time, and the dollar cost of care exhausts the resources of many patients and their families, exacerbating dependency especially for very old patients and in situations, including Alzheimer's disease, in which disease onset is insidious. For chronically ill and disabled older persons as a group, and especially for the very old, there are distinctive problems. As the paper by Barbara Silverstone (in this volume) points out, informal assistance from family and community in caring for the chronically ill is important but may be limited. A realization of the complexity and interrelationships of these issues is essential to anticipating the changing needs of an aging society.

Silverstone writes:

In increasing numbers, very old persons are suffering from chronic mental and physical impairments which demand responses from the social environment extending far beyond conventional short-term interventions. These responses may include ongoing medical, rehabilitative, and skilled nursing attention, help with basic daily chores, and assistance with the more complex financial and bureaucratic negotiations of modern life. [Silverstone, in this volume]

In the view of the committee and its symposium participants, as enunciated by Anne R. Somers (in this volume), "The goal of such care should always be the maximum functional independence . . . of which the patient is capable."

It is important to be clear about this. Maximum functional independence is not a guaranteed money-saver. There is no certainty that a chronically ill person's ability to function relatively independently, whether at home or in an institution, costs less or more in dollars than the alternative. Rather, as the Joint American Medical Association–American Nurses' Association (1983) Task Force to Address the Improvement of Health Care of the Aged Chronically Ill declared in its recent report, "A sense of purpose and control over one's life is integral to the health of the aged. Health care for this group must be oriented toward the individual's self-management."

Most of the very old individuals who are chronically ill and disabled are especially vulnerable to being forced by their financial and other circumstances into dependency. In his paper, David L. Rabin (in this volume) comments: "There is a significant and growing proportion of the population aged 85 and over. It is this group of frail 'old old' who have multiple morbidity combined with a complex of social needs. They also have low and declining incomes and are least able to meet health care costs."

With few exceptions, Medicare does not cover long-term care. Any consideration of these issues, Somers warned, must recognize this void. Rabin cites 1981 median personal income figures of $7,512 for those 65 and over—with the median declining from

$9,780 for those aged 65 to 67 to $4,820 for those 80 and over. (In part these are age-cohort phenomena relating to changing Social Security and pension benefits.) Census data for the 65 + group, not broken out by age, show somewhat lower income as of March 1982 (Table 4). (Income for older people can be expected to change, but how much and in what direction are not clear.) Rabin noted that the typical premium for medigap insurance in 1982 was between $300 and $400, and rates have increased since then by up to 27 percent per year.

Accordingly, changing needs for long-term care, ideally directed toward fostering maximum functional independence, have to be examined from the standpoints of medical prospects, health and social services, changing family structure, and the changing financial situation.

MEDICAL ASPECTS AND PROSPECTS

It is increasingly evident that functional decline is not an inevitable and irreversible concomitant of aging. It does occur, however, and the symposium looked at current biomedical and

TABLE 4   Income, Individuals Aged 65 and Over in the U.S. Civilian Noninstitutionalized Populuation and in the Armed Forces Living on Post or with Their Families Off Post, March 1982

Income	Thousands of Individuals	Percent of Total
Total	25,230	100.0
Without income	283	1.1
$1–$3,999	7,241	28.7
$4,000–$4,999	3,026	12.0
$5,000–$5,999	2,492	9.9
$6,000–$6,999	1,881	7.5
$7,000–$8,499	2,149	8.5
$8,500–$9,999	1,710	6.8
$10,000–$12,499	1,929	7.6
$12,500–$17,499	2,123	8.4
$17,500–$24,999	1,227	4.9
$25,000 +	1,170	4.6

SOURCE: U.S. Department of Commerce. 1983. Bureau of the Census. Current Population Reports, Special Studies, Series P-23, No. 130. Population Profile of the United States: 1982. Washington, D.C.: U.S. Government Printing Office.

epidemiologic research, seeking implications for care of chronically ill older persons in an aging society.

Life expectancy for an infant born in the United States today is about 71 years for males, 78 for female. It has been suggested that the natural human life span ranges between 85 and 110 years; however, controversy about the length of the natural human life span suggests the need for more research. More important for health care planning is knowledge of the years of independent function, and questions of the incidence and causes of dysfunction. Sidney Katz and colleagues developed the Activities of Daily Living Index (relating to bathing, eating, continence, and mobility, for example), now in wide use to describe functionality. The paper by Katz, Greer, Beck, Branch, and Spector (in this volume) carries the idea further, proposing the concept of active life expectancy—independence in the activities of daily living—as being much more useful than conventional life expectancy as a framework for anticipating the health status of the older population.

Although the incidence of chronic illness in the United States increases with age, most older Americans are strikingly active. Fewer than 20 percent of the population aged 75 to 84 and fewer than 50 percent of the 85-and-over group are limited in the activities of daily living. Still, over 6 percent of the 75 to 84 age group and about a quarter of the 85-and-over group are in nursing homes; their numbers are large, and, as might be expected, most of the nursing home resident population is limited in normal activity (Tables 2 and 3). Study of a noninstitutionalized population in Massachusetts by Katz et al. found an active life expectancy of 10 years for those in the 65 to 70 age category and 2.9 years for those 85 and older, with lower active life expectancy for the poor.

The numbers and various biomedical findings run counter to long-held ideas about human aging. In a paper for the 1982 annual meeting of the Institute of Medicine, James F. Fries pointed to the beginning of a "compression of morbidity," caused by the fact that the age at which manifestations of aging and chronic disease first appear is rising faster than life expectancy is increasing. The changing morbidity curve "represents, in many ways, a social ideal—a long, vigorous life culminating, as in Oliver Wendell Holmes' One-Hoss Shay . . . , with a sudden terminal collapse; vitality until the end, and death coming without fear or fury at the natural end of the individual life span."

Fries wrote:

It will not happen this way, of course. . . . Increasing birth cohorts will continue to discharge ever larger numbers of individuals into the older age groups until equilibrium is reached after some 50 years, and the problems we have been experiencing will grow worse before they grow better. Clinical observation for our most vital older citizens suggests a usual terminal decline of months to even a few years, not an abrupt collapse as that of the one-hoss shay. But the compression of morbidity is an achievable phenomenon; it is already occurring in some areas, and it can be made to grow importantly. . . . But the many problems of our increasingly elderly populations continue . . . and require vigorous attack from many directions. . . . [Fries, 1983]

There is a counterview which suggests that the incidence of chronic disease may not decline and that, with prolonged survival, the burden of long-term care will therefore increase. These differing views have been well described in papers by Fries, Myers, and Manton, and by Schneider and Brody (see Bibliography and References). The papers in the present report do not suggest that cases of chronic dysfunction can be expected to decrease or remain stable over the next decades as the numbers of much older people increase. In fact, even with good prevention and the postponement of the onset of chronic disease, the increase in the number of older persons suggests there will be a larger burden of disease overall. The papers do suggest, with powerful implications for both research and long-term care, that (1) as people age into their 80s (at least), dysfunction is far more likely a product of pathology, including social pathology, than of aging; and (2) style of life and style of care can be major determinants of health status.

Cardiovascular performance is one example. Edward G. Lakatta has been studying aging and atherosclerosis, a condition that can begin at a young age. Hidden, subclinical atherosclerosis is widespread and compounds the problem of discerning possible effects of age alone on cardiovascular output.

Smoking, diet, and behavior are associated with clinical manifestations of coronary heart disease and stroke, but quantification and measurement are difficult.

Although the benefits of "chronic exercise" are not known, Lakatta writes that "it is known . . . that the average daily level of physical activity has a marked impact on cardiovascular function." He states:

In the absence of cardiovascular disease [the body's] needs [from the system] are *efficiently* met, nothing more, nothing less. With exercise, cardiac, respiratory, and tissue metabolic systems all increase their level of function from that in the resting state. . . . [B]ed rest can cause up to 40 percent reduction in maximum output and . . . this can be reversed by regular physical activity. Because the . . . conditioning effect can be so great, in studies which attempt to investigate to what extent a disease or an "aging process" alters cardiovascular function . . . the physical activity status must either be controlled for, or considered when interpreting the results. [Lakatta, in this volume]

Reduced activity with age "is likely to be greater in chronically institutionalized subjects," which "might seriously hamper the interpretation of studies which have sought to define an age effect in institutionalized populations."

When marked declines in cardiac output are observed in elderly subjects between 55 and 80 . . . , causes other than age, such as occult coronary disease or physical deconditioning, must be seriously considered to account for the decline. Our greatest challenge . . . in order to preserve cardiac function in advanced age is not to find a "cure" for biologic aging, but rather to prevent physical deconditioning and especially to understand and conquer atherosclerotic vascular disease. . . . [I]nvestigation must begin at an early age, because while this process becomes manifest in middle to late life, it begins much earlier. [Lakatta, in this volume]

Research into cognitive performance shows changes with age, but variation among individuals is considerable. In his paper, Robert Katzman reports that "at age 80, about half of the population is still cognitively 'normal,' " and some people in their 80s and 90s "may be extraordinarily productive . . . ," yet "a significant proportion of individuals in their 80s and 90s develop serious diseases of the brain" that "can lead to progressive loss of cognitive processes to the point where individuals become completely dependent, lose their identity as individuals, and become 'true geriatric tragedies.' " Differentiating among natural aging and age-dependent and other diseases as causal factors is difficult, and here, too, occult disease can contaminate studies.

Mild forgetfulness and slowing of reactions as people reach their 70s and 80s are observed commonly and in test settings; Katzman's paper describes a loss of nerve cells in the brain and a slowing of brain processing in the course of aging. The mechanisms are not fully understood.

The major role, however, is played by disease. Dementia (the term "chronic organic brain syndrome" was used between 1952 and 1980), a severe loss of intellectual ability, is a complex of symptoms of one or more of several diseases. Multi-infarct dementia (from multiple strokes in which vascular occlusions destroy from 50 to 100 grams of brain tissue in the cerebral hemisphere) has been found to account for 20 percent of cases of dementia in the 1960s and 1970s, but its prevalence is decreasing with the decreasing incidence of stroke. Katzman believes Alzheimer's disease is responsible for at least 55 percent of all cases of dementia; another 10 percent of cases involve a mixture of Alzheimer's and multi-infarct dementia.

Individuals with mild to moderate impairment who can function in the community constitute about 10 percent of the over-65 population, according to the clinical literature; from 4 to 5 percent of persons 65 to 84 are victims of severe dementia and can no longer live independently. Severe dementia affects between 15 to 20 percent of the 85-and-over population. Again, the numbers show a mostly healthy older population but a sizable problem nonetheless.

Alzheimer's disease—a disorder of insidious onset and unknown cause that at present is incurable—warrants special concern. Katzman states:

With over 600,000 individuals severely afflicted in the United States and requiring either nursing home care or its equivalent in the community, and with another estimated million individuals in earlier phases of the disorder, the importance of the disease becomes apparent. . . . With the incidence of . . . 3 percent per year in individuals in their mid-80s and with the rapid increase in individuals at risk . . . there is every expectation that Alzheimer's disease will become even more important as a health problem. [Katzman, in this volume]

Katzman stresses the importance of differential diagnosis for the dementias. Experience with follow-up of people who have taken a mental status test shows that it is now possible to identify 80-year-olds in early stages of dementia. Identifying persons with treatable dementias, Katzman observes, would permit recoup of diagnostic costs, result in substantial savings for families (who take care of more than half of all end-stage dementia patients), and reduce nursing home occupancy.

"The tacit assumption in our society that everyone will eventually become 'senile' must be put aside," Katzman says. "The expected norm should be that of a vigorous, intellectually active aging process. Productive years could be increased well past current arbitrary retirement ages for many."

The dementias, as Dan Blazer observes in his paper, are sometimes confused with depressive illness, which itself is often confused with transient depressive symptoms. Unlike occasional depression, most depressive illness is severe, long-lasting, and unexplainable by life's events (although some studies suggest that depressive illness can at times be explained by life's events).

Depressive illness, which "may contribute to significantly decreased functioning in older persons" and may be life-threatening, is "relatively frequent" in later life. The suicide rate among individuals 85 and over is high. Depression is a "severe, but potentially treatable" problem, and, Blazer emphasizes, "must not be assumed to coalesce with the process of aging." Depressive symptoms apparently increase with age; major depressive disorders do not.

As with the dementias, differential diagnosis for depressive illness is particularly important. A biologically driven depression, Blazer notes, is not likely to be addressed successfully by psychosocial intervention. The condition has to be distinguished from schizophrenia. Early-stage dementias are sometimes overlooked in favor of a diagnosis of depression. The problem is complicated by inadequate knowledge of the epidemiology of depressive illness and by the inadequacy of diagnostic tests. Blazer also cautions:

Intoxication with medications, usually prescribed by physicians, frequently leads to depressive symptoms in older persons. . . .
. . . "Learned helplessness" . . . is perhaps the best known behavioral model of depression. . . . Older persons may be at greater risk than individuals at other stages of the life cycle for being placed in situations in which their own behavior apparently has little effect on the behavior of other persons. This is especially true when physical health or cognitive functioning has been inaccurately assessed or when treatment interventions have been prescribed which are restrictive and preclude consultation with the older person. [Blazer, in this volume]

SERVICES AND MISMATCHES

Chronic illness and dysfunction require long-term care, whether in the home, community, or in an institution. Sustained heroic measures to stave off imminent death may be required for the relatively few patients in prolonged danger, and emergencies can develop because of problems in the care of chronically ill individuals. However, the vast majority of individuals in need of long-term care are those whose illnesses and circumstances are not life-threatening in a medical sense but who nevertheless must have help to survive; at increasing ages they are increasingly vulnerable, medically (Tables 2 and 3) and financially (Table 4).

Long-term care is not an alternative to cure. As Fries noted and as Somers observes in her paper, the idea of "cure vs. care" is a false dichotomy, institutionalized in the restrictions of financing programs but unreal as a practical matter. Care beyond the episode-of-illness criteria for Medicare coverage may be for needed recuperation, for recovery over a longer period, or for the remainder of the patient's life. The prognosis is rarely certain.

Long-term care is variously given—formally and informally, at home, in institutions, and may involve family, friends, neighbors, and health care and social service professionals, paraprofessionals, and support staff. If it is to foster the patient's maximum functional capability, long-term care must address a multiplicity of needs—not only logistical and medical but psychological and social as well. It is, in a word, personal. The primary continuing need, as Somers says, is for less intensive care, generally for at least six months and sometimes for years, involving a mix of medical and social services, with maximum realistic involvement of family, neighbors, and other volunteers, as well as formal care.

Information on the extent and distribution of chronic illness and dysfunction is limited and the base for assessing current and future needs for long-term care is consequently inadequate, although information in hand shows serious problems. Data on mental health status suggest sizable numbers but are inconsistent. Neurologic and mental disorders are (1) difficult to ascertain by survey and (2) little surveyed. The latest national nursing home data are old but indicative of the U.S. subpopulation that in 1977 was, it can only be presumed, most in need of long-term care. The primary diagnosis for the largest fraction of nursing home resident patients 65 or older was disease of the circulatory system, 43.8 percent; the second ranking general diagnostic category in the older nursing home population was mental disorders and senility without psychosis, 16.4 percent. Other primary diagnoses accounted for 33.1 percent, and for 6.7 percent the primary diagnosis was unknown.

Silverstone looks at informal supports for chronically ill and dysfunctional older persons, finds them very important although limited, and arrives at a mixed judgment: there is a need to understand the informal system and its potential; the plunge into nursing homes has helped some families and hurt others; and sophisticated case management systems, entailing multiple service referrals, might miss the mark. Personal experiences reveal that the needs of older persons may change very rapidly or that high turnover of personnel employed to provide some services are problems for a case management system. A critical evaluation of such systems is therefore timely.

Current findings suggest that older people who receive home care services experience greater life satisfaction. There are conflicting views of the relative dollar costs of home and institutional care. Exploitative, aggressive behavior between helpless frail elders and their care-givers has long been recognized in nursing homes and is beginning to be seen in families, Silverstone says. On balance:

Informal supports, especially the family, are critical to the survival of many elderly in the community, given the gaps in community services and . . . knowledge about the larger context of informal relationships. . . . But the quality of life for impaired elders over time is not known, nor are the long-range effects on families. Little is known about the strengths and skills of families who do manage well, knowledge which could be tapped for helping other families. [Silverstone, in this volume]

There is, as Somers says, an extensive, expensive long-term care industry in the United States, and its predominant manifestation is the nursing home, which she sees as an interesting, important, but unstable compromise between the Medicare emphasis on short-term, post-hospital recuperation and rehabilitation and the Medicaid emphasis on low-cost, custodial care.

Nursing homes are not necessarily oriented toward maximum functional independence of their patients. Bruce C. Vladeck's Twentieth Century Fund study reported:

The increasingly small proportion of truly horrible nursing homes may be less distressing in the aggregate . . . than the quality of life in the thousands that meet the minimal public standards of adequacy. In these, residents live out the last of their days in an enclosed society without privacy, dignity, or pleasure, subsisting on minimally palatable diets, multiple sedatives, and large doses of television—eventually dying, one suspects, at least partially of boredom. [Vladeck, 1980]

According to the last National Nursing Home Survey data on drugs used in nursing homes, for the period 1973–1974, nearly half of the country's nursing-home patients were receiving tranquilizers and more than a third were receiving hypnotic-sedatives (Table 5).

The nursing home, as Somers observes, typically is set up as if it were a small hospital, but it is not a hospital. Nor, for many resident patients, is it a real home. There is increasing discussion of case management, but questions arise concerning both responsibility for medical and social services and possible conflict between case managers' responsibilities to their agencies and their clients. In any event, Rabin reports, each provider has different incentives and techniques, information and communication are not reimbursable, care teams are rare, and there is no mechanism to encourage professionals to cooperate to meet the

TABLE 5 Number and Percent of Nursing Home Residents, by Type of Medication Received, United States, 1973–1974

Medication Type	Number	Percent
Patients receiving at least one medication	890,000	95.9
Tranquilizers	492,600	47.7
Hypnotic-sedatives	355,200	34.4
Stool softeners	359,500	34.8
Antidepressants	91,300	8.9
Antihypertensives	119,900	11.6
Diuretics	296,700	28.8
Analgesics	377,500	36.6
Diabetic agents	102,000	9.9
Antiinflammatory agents	80,300	7.8
Antiinfectives	91,500	8.9
Antianginal drugs	47,500	4.6
Cardiac glycosides	270,900	26.3
Anticoagulants	12,100	1.2
Vitamins or iron	388,400	37.6
Other	477,300	46.3
None	43,800	—

SOURCE: U.S. Department of Health and Human Services. 1981. National Center for Health Statistics, Public Health Service. Vital and Health Statistics, Data from the National Health Survey, Series 13, No. 51. Hing, E. Characteristics of Nursing Home Residents, Health Status, and Care Received: National Nursing Home Survey, United States, May–December 1977. Hyattsville, Md.: National Center for Health Statistics; DHHS Publication (PHS) 81-1712.

needs of the patient at an acceptable and predictable price. In Somers's opinion:

What is badly needed . . . is recognition . . . that . . . both institutional and noninstitutional modalities are needed and appropriate in given situations, depending partly on the level and duration of care needed, partly on the availability of family and other informal supports; that neither patients nor their care-givers should be locked into any one modality; and that some way must be found . . . that will make possible the most cost-effective, as well as health-effective, use of all our . . . resources. [Somers, in this volume]

Mental illness, the dementias, and their multiple causes and symptoms present distinctive problems. Differential diagnosis is difficult and sometimes unattempted; the mix of medical and psychological services needed is not always clear; and individuals in need of long-term care for mental disorders get such care variously in their communities, in mental hospitals, in nursing homes, or not at all.

The overwhelming influences on trends in long-term care have been the absence of Medicare coverage and the role of Medicaid, with its eligibility restrictions, as well as a general lack of professional interest. It is in this respect, as both Somers and Rabin stress, that the most visible conflict between purposes and programs for long-term care has emerged.

If Medicaid patients are poor enough and are permanently institutionalized in a nursing home, their total costs are paid, Rabin points out. This has encouraged the elderly to spend down all their assets until they are impoverished.

The last National Nursing Home Survey found public assistance, primarily Medicaid, to be the primary source of payment for more than half the resident patients; Medicaid was the primary payment source for 47.8 percent (Table 6).

Increasing medical indigency among chronically ill and disabled older Americans has exacerbated dependency. Somers observes:

If the goal . . . is maximum functional independence for the chronically disabled patient, then the incentives to the system and to individual professionals should be continued improvement, rehabilitation, and the prevention of acute episodes—not just meeting them when the need arises, in at least some cases precisely because continuing care was denied. . . .

TABLE 6 U.S. Nursing Home Residents' Primary Sources of Payment, 1977

Primary Payment Source	Ages									
	<65		65–74		75–84		85+		Total	
	Number	%	Number	%	Number	%	Number	%	Number	%
All sources	177,100	100.0	211,400	100.0	464,700	100.0	449,900	100.0	1,303,100	100.0
Own income or family support	46,500	26.2	70,800	33.5	201,900	43.4	181,700	40.4	500,900	38.4
Medicare	1,300[a]	0.8	6,200	3.0	11,900	2.6	6,800	1.5	26,200	2.0
Medicaid	92,500	52.2	107,900	51.8	204,000	43.9	218,700	48.6	623,300	47.8
Other government assistance or welfare	22,400	12.7	14,900	7.1	23,000	4.9	23,100	5.1	83,400	6.4
Other sources[b]	14,300	8.1	11,400	5.4	23,900	5.1	19,600	4.4	69,200	5.3

NOTE: Because of rounding, figures may not add to totals.

[a]Figure does not meet standards of reliability or precision.

[b]Including religious organizations, volunteer agencies, Veterans Administration contracts, initial payment for life-care funds, and instances of no charge.

SOURCE: U.S. Department of Health and Human Services. 1981. National Center for Health Statistics, Public Health Service. Vital and Health Statistics, Series 13, No. 51. Hing, E. Characteristics of Nursing Home Residents, Health Status, and Care Received: National Nursing Home Survey, United States, May–December 1977. Hyattsville, Md.: National Center for Health Statistics; DHHS Publication (PHS) 81-1712.

[There] is the basic conflict . . . between a welfare program and the goal of . . . maximum functional independence. By limiting eligibility to those who are already seriously dependent . . . medically and financially . . . or to those who make themselves dependent for this purpose . . . the program not only fails to encourage independent functioning but actually promotes dependency of both types. . . . [Somers, in this volume]

Mismatches are clear. And Katz et al. note:

Currently, efforts in [disease] prevention deal mostly with primary and secondary prevention, i.e., averting diseases, injuries, or defects, and early detection of disease. Much less attention is focused on tertiary prevention, that is, efforts to improve residual function, to prevent the progression of disability, and to improve the quality of life. The balance in the focus of health policies between these types of prevention should be changed toward a greater emphasis on tertiary prevention in view of the aging of the population, the increasing importance of chronic diseases, and the high cost of long-term care. . . . [N]ecessary changes in current health policies are hampered by the absence of sound information about the functional determinants of health and the functional outcomes of services. . . . Health policy could increasingly take into account the uniqueness of problems of and services for the elderly. [Katz et al., in this volume]

CONCLUSIONS AND RECOMMENDATIONS

Demographic, epidemiologic, biomedical, economic, and social findings point to an emerging, substantial challenge to health care and related service for chronically ill older persons in the United States. The increasing older population will include—as more people reach the age ranges for chronic illness—a larger number of individuals in need of extended care to help them function as independently as is medically possible. The challenge to biomedical, social, and behavioral research in this regard is manifest—pursuit of studies to prevent and alleviate the burden—but scientific advances come sporadically, unpredictably, and never soon enough. Questions about long-term care face the nation as a whole; these are issues of values and of policy for which the research base also is inadequate. At present there does not appear to be a good match between the needs of older persons for extended care and the available care. Furthermore, as the population ages, these disparities will worsen and intensify pressures for the equitable allocation of services to the population as a whole.

The committee notes that studies and surveys consistent with some of its recommendations have begun or are in planning; the committee's recommendations in these regards are intended to place the importance of such efforts in perspective and to endorse their continuing support. Several areas of study recommended by the committee will require the determination of research agendas and priorities.

The Emerging Older Population

As the population of the United States ages, the country can expect both a much larger population of older people who are generally healthy and significantly increased numbers of individuals suffering from chronic, disabling conditions. Active life expectancy appears to extend well into the 70s. Currently, the proportion of persons with chronic illness and dysfunction begins to rise in the middle years, increasing markedly in the mid-70s and sharply in the mid-80s. Although older Americans of the future are expected to be financially better off than their predecessors as private pension plans take effect, by today's standards the income of most older people is very low, especially for those in their 80s and over. Age cohorts differ, and it is dangerous to assume that the future will not differ from the past either for better or for worse. Studies of the emerging older population have begun and will be of considerable importance in health planning.

The committee recommends:

• frequent periodic survey and timely publication of statistical data on the physical and mental health and functional status of the entire U.S. population, with detailed information for age groups perhaps in 3- or 5-year intervals, and with subpopulations identified by ethnic group and by type and duration of health care and related services, type of living settings, method of payment, and pertinent economic factors (the National Research Council Committee on National Statistics has begun a study of needs for statistical information on the health of older persons);

• examination of the social and economic costs of chronic illness and dysfunction and how those might best be met. These issues are being carefully examined in the planning effort on alternative approaches to long-term care.

Disease and Dysfunction

Research increasingly suggests that dysfunction is a consequence not of aging, at least into the 80s, but of pathology, and it is becoming clearer that style of life and care can affect health status (see Lakatta, in this volume). Although many changes do occur with aging, fewer than half the over-85 population are limited in the basic activities of daily living (although they may be limited in other functions), and such limitation is not necessarily attributable to aging.

In no small measure, the decline of heart disease, cerebral vascular disease, and arteriosclerosis has contributed to the expansion of the older population. Recent studies of cardiovascular performance in the approximately 50 percent of older persons free of heart disease show no demonstrable age effect. Bed rest can cause up to a 40 percent reduction in cardiac output, but this effect is reversible by regular activity.

Cognitive performance changes with age, but variation among individuals is considerable, and at least half the population at age 80 shows little or no decline in cognitive function. There is minor fall-off in short-term memory and brain processing speed, but diseases underlie the dementias, some treatable if the differential diagnosis is made. To repeat Katzman's assertion, eventually our society will have to relinquish its unspoken assumption that all people become "senile" as they age.

Alzheimer's disease is an expanding tragedy: a degenerative, devastating brain disease afflicting over 600,000 middle-aged and older people in the United States; an incidence of 3 percent in people in their mid-80s; an increasing population at risk; cause and cure both unknown; and a heavy burden of care.

Depressive illness, other mental illness, transient depressions, and the dementias can be confused, and accurate differential diagnosis can mean the difference between recovery and prolonged dysfunction. Depression leading to dysfunction may be a consequence of the nature of care: intoxication with medications can induce depression, as can inaccurate assessment and inappropriate treatment of physical health or cognitive function of a patient unable to affect the behavior of other people, including health care providers.

The diseases reviewed in this volume by no means constitute a comprehensive list. Cancer, arthritis, diabetes, digestive diseases, and others are of no less concern. Mental illness tends to be neglected as an aspect of long-term care. For the most part, causes of dysfunction are not understood sufficiently, and current data on health status as well as projected estimates of epidemiologic trends are insufficient.

The committee recommends:

• increased research to distinguish the effects of disease and social and cultural factors from the effects of aging;

• increased effort to conceptualize and measure active life expectancy;

• increased research into the causes, prevalence, distribution, and prevention of and rehabilitative treatment for chronic diseases and dysfunction;

• increased effort to expand possibilities for rehabilitation and reversal of effects of diseases associated with aging;

• accelerated research on the dementias and on all aspects of Alzheimer's disease, and accelerated development of differential diagnostic techniques for the dementias and symptoms of mental illness.

Long-Term Care

Long-term care has been a chronic misfit in U.S. health care and social service programs. There is no social consensus on either its definition or purposes. Considered custodial and therefore outside the medical mainstream, as Somers observes, long-term care for other than the relatively few older disabled people who are financially secure has evolved as an inadequate and in many ways self-defeating welfare program (with dependence as the admission ticket) in medical garb. With their needs for long-term care generally excluded from Medicare (a medical program) and with their resources dwindling, the unfortunate sequence for many older, chronically ill people in the United States has been spending down in order to qualify for welfare programs, chiefly Medicaid, followed by irreversible exacerbation of dependency. There has been insufficient emphasis on rehabilitation or reversal of debilitating effects.

Exclusion of long-term care from Medicare may have been purposeful. The result, the consignment of an expanding number of older people into a welfare population and the consequent quasi-medicalization of this growing welfare problem as the alternative to abandonment, has occurred by default.

The American Medical Association–American Nurses' Association (1983) Task Force found "provision of care to the chronically ill aged . . . inadequate" and that current funding mechanisms "serve as barriers to effective and organized care." The task force recommended that "extensive research efforts on new health care systems [including demonstration projects combining housing, health care, and social services] for the aged" be analyzed in detail, perhaps by the Institute of Medicine of the National Academy of Sciences.

There are concerns as well that debilitating effects of disease in older persons may be regarded as inevitable and irreversible, and that such attitudes toward aging, disease prevention, and prospects for rehabilitation can become self-fulfilling prophecies. Clearly, diagnosis and treatment for chronic illness and dysfunction and both the nature and financing of long-term care and treatment have to be evaluated in terms of their effects on patients and their implications for the aging U.S. society.

The committee recommends:

• a major study of U.S. public policy and resources for long-term health care and related services for chronic illness and dysfunction, including evaluation of demonstration projects combining housing, social, and health services, and taking into account the country's changing age distribution, the needs of older persons, and the financing of long-term care (the Institute of Medicine has begun planning such a study);

• study of factors affecting quality and outcomes of nursing home care (the Institute of Medicine has undertaken a broad study of regulation and measurement of the quality of nursing home life and care);

• study—including longitudinal tracking of individual patients—of the outcomes of various types and combinations of long-term care for chronic illness and dysfunction in all age groups, with special attention to middle age and later years;

• study to develop measurable units of long-term care efficiency, to better assess the value of different services;

• study of attitudes and assumptions of patients, their families, and of health care and social service professionals and support staff toward aging, and study of the influences of expectations on disease prevention, treatment, and outcomes.

National Need

The committee feels that the nation's attention urgently needs to be directed to the implications of the aging of our society for long-term care for chronically ill and dysfunctional older persons. This summary and the following papers recommend numerous, needed studies—to enable us to understand, diagnose, treat, and, where possible, prevent or reverse the effects of chronic illness, and to meet the nation's needs for long-term care. The United States can take pride in its healthier older population, but the country has not sufficiently addressed the growing burden of chronic illness and dysfunction and its consequences for using and allocating health care resources.

BIBLIOGRAPHY AND REFERENCES

American Medical Association and American Nurses' Association. 1983. Report of the Joint AMA/ANA Task Force to Address the Improvement of Health Care of the Aged Chronically Ill. Issued at Kansas City, Missouri. April 5, 1983.

Ansak, M. L., and R. Lindheim. 1983. On Lok: Housing and Adult Day Health Care for the Frail Elderly. Berkeley: Center for Environmental Design Research, College of Environmental Design, University of California at Berkeley.

Burke, R. E., and B. D. Dunlop. 1981. Analysis of the Impact of Government Programs on Long-Term Care Services: Description of the Long-Term Care System. Report to the American Health Care Association. Cambridge, Mass.: ABT Associates Inc.

Butler, L. H., and P. W. Newacheck. 1981. Health and social factors relevant to long-term-care policy. In Meltzer, J., F. Farrow, and H. Richman, eds. Policy Options in Long-Term Care. Chicago: University of Chicago Press.

Covell, R. M. 1980. The impact of regulation on health care quality. In Leven, A., ed. Regulating Health Care: The Struggle for Control. Proceedings of The Academy of Political Sciences 33(4):111-125.

Farrow, F., T. Joe, J. Meltzer, and H. Richman. 1981. Introduction: The framework and directions for change. In Meltzer, J., F. Farrow, and H. Richman, eds. Policy Options in Long-Term Care. Chicago: University of Chicago Press.

Feldman, J. J. 1983. Work ability of the aged under conditions of improving mortality. Milbank Memorial Fund Quarterly, Health and Society 61:430-444.

Fries, J. F. 1983. The compression of morbidity. Milbank Memorial Fund Quarterly, Health and Society 61:397-419.

Fries, J. F. 1984. The compression of morbidity: Miscellaneous comments about a theme. The Gerontologist 24:354-359.

Hahn, H. 1984. The Issue of Equality: European Perceptions of Unemployment for Disabled Persons. New York: World Rehabilitation Fund.

Hynes, C. J. 1980. The regulation of nursing homes: A case study. In Levin, A., ed. Regulating Health Care: The Struggle for Control. Proceedings of The Academy of Political Science 33(4):126-136.

Levin, A., ed. 1980. Regulating Health Care: The Struggle for Control. Proceedings of The Academy of Political Science, Vol. 33, No. 4.

Meltzer, J., F. Farrow, and H. Richman, eds. 1981. Policy Options in Long-Term Care. Chicago: University of Chicago Press.

Meyers, G. C., and K. G. Manton. 1984. Compression of mortality: Myth or reality? The Gerontologist 24:346-353.

National Research Council and Institute of Medicine. Forthcoming. Committee on an Aging Society. The Aging Society: Older Persons, Productive Lives. Washington: National Academy Press.

Quinn, J. B. 1984. Staying ahead: Life-care centers could prove risky to your old-age security. Washington Post, May 14, 1984.

Rice, D. P., and J. J. Feldman. 1983. Living longer in the United States: Demographic changes and health needs of the elderly. Milbank Memorial Fund Quarterly, Health and Society 61:362-396.

Scanlon, W. J., and J. Feder. 1984. The long-term care marketplace: An overview. Health-care Financial Management, January.

Schneider, E. L., and J. A. Brody. 1983. Aging, natural death, and the compression of morbidity: Another view. New England Journal of Medicine 309:854-856.

Somers, A. R. 1982. Long-term care for the elderly and disabled: A new health priority. New England Journal of Medicine 307:221-226.

Somers, A. R., and D. R. Fabian, eds. 1981. The Geriatric Imperative; An Introduction to Gerontology and Clinical Geriatrics. New York: Appleton Century Croft.

U.S. Congress. 1984. House of Representatives. Select Committee on Aging. The Economics of Aging: A Need for Preretirement Planning. Hearing, September 16, 1983. 98th Cong., 1st sess. Washington, D.C.: U.S. Government Printing Office; Comm. Pub. 98-422.

U.S. Congress. 1984. House of Representatives. Select Committee on Aging. Rising Health Care Costs and the Elderly. Hearing, January 20, 1984. 98th Cong., 2d sess. Washington, D.C.: U.S. Government Printing Office; Comm. Pub. 98-427.

U.S. Congress. 1984. House of Representatives. Select Committee on Aging. Subcommittee on Health and Long-Term Care. Crisis in Health Care: The States' Perspective. Hearing, August 11, 1983. 98th Cong., 1st sess. Washington, D.C.: U.S. Government Printing Office; Comm. Pub. 98-424.

U.S. Congress. 1984. House of Representatives. Select Committee on Aging. Subcommittee on Housing and Consumer Interests. Housing the Elderly: Alternative Options (Erie, Pa.). Hearing, October 17, 1983. 98th Cong., 1st sess. Washington, D.C.: U.S. Government Printing Office; Comm. Pub. 98-421.

U.S. Congress. 1984. Office of Technology Assessment. Medical Technology and Costs of the Medicare Program. Washington, D.C.: Office of Technology Assessment.

U.S. Congress. 1984. Office of Technology Assessment. Technology and Aging in America. Washington, D.C.: Office of Technology Assessment.

U.S. Congress. 1984. Senate. Special Committee on Aging. Developments in Aging: 1983; Vols. 1-2. 98th Cong., 2d sess. Washington, D.C.: U.S. Government Printing Office. Report 98-360.

U.S. Department of Commerce. 1983. Bureau of the Census. Current Population Reports, Special Studies, Series P-23, No. 130. Population Profile of the United States: 1982. Washington, D.C.: U.S. Government Printing Office.

U.S. Department of Health and Human Services. 1980. National Center for Health Statistics, Public Health Service. Vital and Health Statistics, Data from the National Health Survey, Series 10, No. 135. Black, E. R. Use of Special Aids, United States—1977. Hyattsville, Md.: National Center for Health Statistics; DHHS Publication (PHS) 81-1563.

U.S. Department of Health and Human Services. 1981. National Center for Health

Statistics, Public Health Service. Vital and Health Statistics, Data from the National Health Survey, Series 13, No. 51. Hing, E. Characteristics of Nursing Home Residents, Health Status, and Care Received: National Nursing Home Survey, United States, May–December 1977. Hyattsville, Md.: National Center for Health Statistics; DHHS Publication (PHS) 81-1712.

U.S. Department of Health and Human Services. 1981. National Center for Health Statistics, Public Health Service. Vital and Health Statistics, Data from the National Health Survey, Series 13, No. 59. Hing, E., and B. K. Cypress. Use of Health Services by Women 65 Years of Age and Over. United States. Hyattsville, Md.: National Center for Health Statistics; DHHS Publication (PHS) 81-1720.

U.S. Department of Health and Human Services. 1982. National Center for Health Statistics, Public Health Service. Vital and Health Statistics, Series 10, No. 66. Gagnon, R. O., J. E. DeLozier, and T. McLemore. The National Ambulatory Medical Care Survey, United States, 1979 Summary. Hyattsville, Md.: National Center for Health Statistics; DHHS Publication (PHS) 82-1727.

U.S. Department of Health and Human Services. 1982. National Center for Health Statistics, Public Health Service. Vital and Health Statistics, Series 10, No. 141. Bloom, B. Current Estimates from the National Health Interview Survey: United States, 1981. Hyattsville, Md.: National Center for Health Statistics; DHHS Publication (PHS) 82-1569.

U.S. Department of Health and Human Services. 1982. National Institute on Aging, National Institutes of Health, Public Health Service. Toward an Independent Old Age: A National Plan for Research on Aging. Bethesda, Md.: National Institutes of Health; NIH Publication No. 82-2453.

U.S. Department of Health and Human Services. 1983. National Center for Health Statistics, Public Health Service. Gardocki, G. J. Utilization of Outpatient Care Resources. Hyattsville, Md.: National Center for Health Statistics; DHHS Publication (PHS) 83-1240.

U.S. Department of Health and Human Services. 1983. National Center for Health Statistics, Public Health Service. Prevalence of published chronic conditions, rates by sex and age: United States, 1981. Unpublished data from the National Health Interview Survey. March 31, 1983.

U.S. Department of Health and Human Services. 1983. National Center for Health Statistics, Public Health Service. Feller, B. A. Americans Needing Help to Function at Home. Advance Data From Vital and Health Statistics No. 92. Hyattsville, Md.: National Center for Health Statistics; DHHS Publication No. (PHS)83-1250.

U.S. Department of Health and Human Services. 1983. National Center for Health Statistics, Public Health Service. Vital and Health Statistics, Series 10, No. 143. Wilder, C. S. Disability Days: United States, 1980. Hyattsville, Md.: National Center for Health Statistics; DHHS Publication (PHS) 83-1571.

U.S. Department of Health and Human Services. 1983. National Institute on Aging, National Institutes of Health, Public Health Service. Report of the National Advisory Council on Aging: For a National Plan of Research on Aging. Bethesda, Md.: National Institutes of Health.

U.S. Department of Health and Human Services. 1983. National Institute on Aging, National Institutes of Health, Public Health Service. Special Report on Aging 1983. Bethesda, Md.: National Institutes of Health; NIH Publication 83-2489.

U.S. Federal Council on the Aging. 1979. Key Issues in Long Term Care: A Progress Report.

Vladeck, B. C. 1980. Unloving Care: The Nursing Home Tragedy. New York: Basic Books.

Waxing of the Gray, Waning of the Green

David L. Rabin*

The aging of our society is predictable. The consequences of an ever-increasing number of elderly, however, guarantee unpredictability as to how health services for the elderly will be financed in the future. Our willingness to finance the current health care system is strained. Recent substantial changes in financing mitigate but do not resolve the problem. They encourage certain types of services while discouraging others. The changes indicate the direction but not the shape of future health services for the aged.

Federal law acknowledged the financial need of the aged for health care by passage of Medicare, Title XVIII of the Social Security Act, in 1965. The title provided financial access to acute health care for the aged. Medicare reflected the reality that many aged could not afford the costs of hospitalization or of private insurance to offset these costs. Medicare successfully provided financial access to acute services for the elderly. Service use increased and the proportion of out-of-pocket expenses the elderly paid for health care decreased. The combination of access to services and the benefits of medical technology may have contributed to the development of a "different" elderly population than

*Professor and Associate Chairman, Department of Community and Family Medicine, School of Medicine, Georgetown University, Washington, D.C.

existed when Medicare began. The aged population now has a different age structure, a changed economic status, and different health care needs. The most significant change is in the number of "old old," where needs are greatest. If we are to continue to meet our existing commitment to the aged in the light of a doubling in that portion of the population by the year 2000, changes in health care financing and services must be made.

To illustrate the problem, this paper highlights demographic data reflecting changes within the aged population and relates these changes to the morbidity of the aged and their service use. Income and insurance coverage of the aged are discussed in the context of recent legislative change in entitlement programs. Implications for fulfilling our commitments to the old old in the light of their emergent needs and also the problems of delivering health care are discussed.

DEMOGRAPHY

We are well aware of the substantial past growth in the elderly population. There has been a 60 percent increase in the number aged 65 and over since 1960 and a 2 percent increase in that proportion of our population.[1] There will be more than a doubling in the number of elderly by the year 2000 from that of 1960 and a further 2 percent increase in the proportion of aged in our total population. Current projections indicate a continuing increase in the number and proportion of the elderly to the year 2050, when a quarter of the population will be over 65.[2] The increases, both in numbers and in the proportion of the elderly, are widely accepted indicators of the graying of our society. Less fully appreciated are changes within the aged population. The 1980 census somewhat unexpectedly revealed a larger number of old old, those 85 +. This has led to important recent revisions in the projected age structure of the elderly. These revisions have major implications for the volume of morbidity with which our health care system will be presented. Table 1 shows changes in the aged population from 1960 to the year 2000. From 1960 to the present there was a slight reduction in the proportion of the population aged 65 to 74 from 66 percent to 61 percent. From now until the year 2000 there will be a further reduction down to 50 percent. In turn, there will be an increase in those aged 75 to 84 to 35 percent of the aged by the year 2000. More significantly, those

TABLE 1   Population of the United States 65 and Over in 1960, 1980, and Projections for 2000: Number and Proportion by Age (in 1,000s)

Age Group	Year		
	1960	1980	2000
Total population 65+			
Number	16,560	25,544	35,036
Percent	9.2	11.3	13.1
65–74			
Number	10,997	15,578	17,693
Percent	66.4	61.0	50.5
75–84			
Number	4,633	7,727	12,207
Percent	28.0	30.2	34.8
85+			
Number	929	2,240	5,136
Percent	5.6	8.8	14.7

SOURCE: Taeuber, C. 1983. America in Transition: An Aging Society. Developments in Aging, 1982, 1:1-41; A Report of the Senate Special Committee on Aging. Washington, D.C.: U.S. Government Printing Office.

85 and above will increase proportionately from about 5 percent of the aged in 1960 to nearly 9 percent in 1980 and to 15 percent by the year 2000. These projections are the recent Bureau of the Census mid-range assumptions of future population. If these assumptions are correct, there will be a substantial increase in a population for whom we have heretofore had little experience and data, that is those 85+, the old old. While the increase in the 85+ population is the most significant aspect of the increase in the aged population, there has also been substantial change even within the age structure of this old old population. Table 2 indicates that those 85+ increased nearly fourfold in number from the year 1950 to 2.3 million in 1980. As with the over-65 population, those old old closest to 85 years of age decreased proportionately from 75 percent in 1950 to 67 percent in 1980. Those 90 to 94, 95 to 99, and 100+ each have increased as a proportion of the elderly over 85, with the proportionate increase greatest for those oldest. Those 100+ have increased threefold and now represent 1 percent of the aged population, numbering 23,000.[3] While the numbers are small, continued accumulation of those "ancient" aged should have an increasing impact on

TABLE 2 Number and Percent of Population 85 and Over for Years 1950, 1960, 1970, and 1980 (in 1,000s)

	Year			
Age Group	1950	1960	1970	1980
Total population, all ages	150,697	179,323	203,212	226,505
85 + population	576	857	1,412	2,264
85–89				
Number	430	649	1,018	1,526
Percent	74.6	75.7	72.1	67.4
90–94				
Number	119	171	313	564
Percent	20.6	19.9	22.1	24.9
95–99				
Number	25	34	73	151
Percent	4.3	4.0	5.2	6.7
100 +				
Number	2	3	8[a]	23
Percent	0.34	0.35	0.56	1.0

[a]100 + population figures revised since 1970 Census. Data for this group are from Seigel, J., and J. Passel. 1976. New estimates of the number of centenarians in the United States. Journal of the American Statistical Association 71:559-566.

SOURCE: 1950 and 1960 data from U.S. Bureau of the Census, 1970 Census of the Population, Characteristics of the Population, 1970; 1, Part 1, Section 1, Table 51. Washington, D.C., U.S. Government Printing Office. 1970 data from ibid., Table 52. 1980 data from Passel, J., Bureau of the Census, personal communication, June 1983.

requirements for health services and government responsibilities, as people outlive their social, familial, and financial resources.

MORTALITY

The growth of the older aged population has occurred as a result of reductions in death rates among the elderly. From 1950 to 1980 mortality declined for all age groups of the aged population.[4] However, reductions in death rates were not proportionate for all ages, as shown in Table 3. In general, increases in the rate of reduction of death rates over time were greater in successive decades, and the greatest overall decline, nearly 30 percent since 1960, was for those 85 and over. The second greatest proportionate decrease in death rates in the past decade was among those 65 to 74, assuring a continued accumulation of the old old for

TABLE 3 Death Rates (per 100,000) of the Population 65 and Over by Age and Percent of Change Over Time for Years 1950, 1960, 1970, 1980[a]

Age	1950	1960	Percent Change	1970	Percent Change	1980[a]	Percent Change	Overall Percent Change
65–74	4,067.7	3,822.1	−4.56	3,582.7	− 6.26	2,968.5	−17.14	−27.02
75–84	9,331.1	8,745.2	−6.28	8,004.4	− 8.47	7,178.4	−10.32	−23.07
85+	20,196.9	19,857.5	−1.68	17,539.4	−11.67	14,489.6	−17.39	−28.26

[a]1980 figures are estimates.

SOURCE: Department of Health and Human Services. 1982. Health—United States, 1982. Hyattsville, Md.: Public Health Service; DHHS Publication No. (PHS)83-1232.

the remainder of the century since those 65 to 74 are the most numerous among the aged.

Crimmins[5] recently commented on projected demographic trends, reviewing recent mortality experience indicating some evidence that mortality rates may actually continue to decrease for age groups above 85. If this is true, continued increases in the ancient old categories seem likely. Taking the Bureau of the Census population projections based on three different assumptions of future mortality in the aged, Crimmins notes that differing assumptions matter little in age structure to the year 2000, except in the continued survivability of those over 85. Under any of the mortality assumptions, the major impact on the age structure of the population will be on the number of old old.

Crimmins analyzed differences in death rates of three age groups above 65 by cause of death for the period 1970 to 1977. The analysis showed that decreases in disease-specific death rates per thousand population for females 85 + were substantially greater than for other old age groups. The decline in death rates for females 85 + was nearly five times greater than for those 65 to 74 and nearly two and a half times greater than for those 75 to 84. The rates of change of death rates for men were lower than for females 75 to 84 and 85 + . The major contributors to the death rate changes for both males and females between 1970 and 1977 were declines in mortality due to heart disease, cerebral vascular disease, and arteriosclerosis.

The mortality assumption made by the Bureau of the Census that death rates will continue to decline at their current pace for the mid-range projections seems reasonable but not certain, at least to the year 2000. This assumption is based on recent experience with declining death rates, primarily from cardiovascular diseases. There is much we do not know about the causes of these diseases and the relationship of declining death rates to therapy or risk factors.[6] Assumptions about future deaths from these diseases are based more on hope than certainty. Based on imperfect knowledge, one must judge which assumptions are more likely if one is to plan for the future.

Table 4 shows 1979 age-specific leading causes of death for the population 65 + .[7] Diseases of the heart account for nearly 45 percent of all deaths. The second and third leading causes of death are malignant neoplasms and cancer and cerebral vascular disease; together they account for an additional 30 percent of deaths.

TABLE 4   Number and Percent of Deaths by 10 Leading Causes
for Population 65 Years and Over, 1979

Cause	Number	Percent
Diseases of heart	566,924	44.6
Malignant neoplasms and cancer	247,922	19.5
Cerebral vascular disease	144,891	11.4
Chronic obstructive pulmonary disease and allied conditions	38,249	3.0
Pneumonia and influenza	36,598	2.9
Atherosclerosis	27,521	2.2
Accidents and adverse effects	24,032	1.9
Diabetes mellitus	23,948	1.9
Nephritis, nephrotic syndrome, and nephrosis	11,966	0.9
Chronic liver disease	8,957	0.7
Total deaths 65 +	1,271,656	100.0

SOURCE: U.S. Department of Health and Human Services. 1982. National Center for Health Statistics, Public Health Service. Final Mortality Statistics, 1979. Monthly Vital Statistics Advance Report, Supplement. Hyattsville, Md.: Public Health Service; DHHS Publication No. (PHS)82-1230.

The three leading causes of death account for three out of every four deaths occurring among the aged. Two of the three, heart disease and stroke, account for much of the recent decrease in death rates; this decrease is associated with increased access to and use of medical services, as provided for under Medicare. For both these disease categories, more effective diagnosis and medical or surgical therapy for the underlying medical conditions of hypertension and arteriosclerosis have become available. It may be assumed that increased use of services has resulted in better treatment of these conditions, with a decrease in the complications of coronary artery and cerebral vascular disease, and has thus contributed in some degree to the decrease in mortality. The improved socioeconomic status of the elderly, noted later, may also be significant.

For those now reaching 65 and succeeding cohorts, mortality rates from heart disease and stroke may decline even further as a result of both additional advances in medical technology and a more favorable experience with known risk factors.[8] Evidence on hypertensive therapy suggests that those now approaching 65 have been more widely treated with antihypertensive medications, putting them less at risk of complications.[9] Complications from all three of the vascular disorders are associated with smoking. Since 1955 there has been a progressive decline in the proportion of persons smoking for the cohort now becoming 65, particularly among males. In 1955, 62 percent of those in the age group 35 to 44 were smokers; by 1975 only 34 percent of males in this cohort still smoked. The incidence of smoking behavior in females also declined.[10] This suggests that the cohort now becoming 65 + may have an even greater decline in mortality in the period beyond age 65 than cohorts becoming 65 in the past. The expectation of continuing decreases in death rates is based on decreases in heart disease, cerebral vascular disease, and arteriosclerosis. Together these cardiovascular diseases account for 50 percent of mortality for those 65 to 69 and 71 percent for those 85 + . Death rates from cancer have remained unchanged and account for 19.5 percent of aged deaths. Further decreases are more conjectural. Recent advances in cell biochemistry and the development of chemotherapeutic agents give rise to cautious optimism that cancer may be more effectively treated, delaying if not preventing cancer deaths in the next 20 years.

MORBIDITY

Age is the single best indicator of morbidity, and morbidity is the single most important determinant of use of health services. Aging of the aged population is a major factor in determining the volume of illness for which the health care system is responsible. Since there was a smaller old old population in the past, small numbers of persons in age groups beyond 65 to 74 were interviewed in National Health Interview surveys, and most national morbidity data were aggregated for the total population 65 + . The morbidity in these older age groups is substantially different from that for 65- to 74-year-olds, the largest group of the elderly. The differences have important implications for future expectations of health care use, particularly for use of services by those with chronic illness with disability. Such persons require long-term care involving social as well as medical services. The prevalence of persons with chronic disabilities as reported in the National Health Interview Survey of the noninstitutionalized population shows dramatic increases in chronic disability with age, as shown in Table 5.[11] Chronic disability is indicated by reporting of a limitation of physical activity, emotional or nervous limitation, some decrease in mobility, or a per-

TABLE 5 Number (in 1,000s) and Percent of Persons With One or More Selected Physical or Emotional Limitations, by Age, 1977[a]

Age	Number	Percent
All ages	29,644	14.0
65+	9,786	44.0
65–74	5,605	39.3
75–84	3,292	49.5
85+	889	65.6

[a]Limitation of activity, emotional or nervous limitation, mobility limitation, or personal care limitations.

SOURCE: U.S. Department of Health and Human Services. National Center for Health Statistics, Public Health Service. Unpublished data from the National Health Interview Survey.

sonal care limitation. The proportion of persons with chronic disabilities is 14 percent for all ages, but increases to 39 percent for those 65 to 74 and to 66 percent for those 85 and over.

The long-term care system is affected to the degree that the chronically disabled need help. Table 6 shows that the rate per thousand of the adult population needing the help of another person dramatically increases with age. While 3 percent of all adults need help from another person because of a chronic health problem, this increases to 44 percent of those 85+. There is a sixfold increase in the proportion needing help, from 7 percent

TABLE 6 Number (in 1,000s) and Percent of Adults Who "Need Help of Another Person" for One or More Selected Activities, by Age, 1979[a]

Age	Total Adults	Percent Needing Help
All adults	153,178	3.17
65–74	14,929	6.99
75+	8,414	21.10
75–84	6,869	16.03
85+	1,544	43.65

[a]Data are based on household interviews of the civilian, noninstitutionalized population.

SOURCE: U.S. Department of Health and Human Services. 1983. National Center for Health Statistics, Public Health Service. Feller, B. A. Americans Needing Help to Function at Home. Advance Data from Vital and Health Statistics, No. 92. Hyattsville, Md.: Public Health Service; DHHS Publication No. (PHS)83-1250.

of those 65 to 74 to 44 percent for those who are 85 + .[12] No age-specific data are available for age categories above 85 +, but it is reasonable to conjecture that the small but proportionately rapidly growing number of persons in these age groups consists of a high proportion of individuals who have exhausted their social and fiscal resources and require long-term care at home or in an institution. Data are also available on the particular kinds of services chronically disabled adults require by age, from questions on the 1979 Home Care Supplement to the National Health Interview Survey. The rate of persons per thousand needing assistance with particular activities is shown in Table 7. The same marked change by age group is apparent, with a nearly sevenfold difference in the need for help between the young aged, 65 to 74, and those 85 + .[12] The percentage varies, but the numbers needing help with every activity, from walking to toileting to eating increases by 700 to 1,000 percent for those over 85 compared with the age group 65 to 74. Need for help in performing these activities indicates the need for personal care from someone who can be in attendance periodically or continually. These numbers relate only to the needs of the noninstitutionalized population.

While disease-specific data are not available for the old old, evidence indicates that a high and increasing proportion of disability and "need for help" is due to the rising prevalence rate of the senile dementias, particularly of the Alzheimer's type. This age-dependent disease, of unknown etiology, can in an otherwise healthy individual devastate the brain and lead to total incapacity. While the prevalence rate of senile dementia among persons aged 65 is only 4 percent, estimates of its incidence in those surviving beyond age 80 range from 17 to 30 percent.[13–16] "Pseudodementias," related to the high incidence of depression and other mental disorders, also increase with age.[17]

In 1977, 23 percent of those 85 + were residing in nursing homes, usually with multiple physical and social impairments.[18] It is estimated that 55 to 60 percent of nursing home residents suffer from senile dementia or other mental disorders,[19] but the evidence implies that the majority of those with severe dementia are being cared for in the community.[13] The data therefore demonstrate the substantial and increasing need for care for the old old population, which must be provided both at home and in institutions.

TABLE 7 Rate (per 1,000) of Aged Persons Who Need Help in Basic Physical Activities and by Type of Activity and Age, 1979[a]

Age	Needs Help in One or More Basic Activities	Walking	Going Outside	Bathing	Dressing	Using Toilet	Getting In or Out of Chair	Eating
All adults	22.5	16.1	13.7	9.1	7.1	5.5	4.9	2.0
65–74	52.6	39.2	34.2	20.4	14.4	11.6	9.0	3.9
75+	157.0	115.9	109.3	73.1	48.3	42.3	34.5	13.8
75–84	114.0	83.6	73.5	50.7	32.9	28.4	25.8	8.4
85+	348.4	259.7	268.8	172.9	116.6	104.9	72.5	37.6

[a]Data are based on household interviews of the civilian, noninstitutionalized population.

SOURCE: U.S. Department of Health and Human Services. 1983. National Center for Health Statistics, Public Health Service. Feller, B. A. Americans Needing Help to Function at Home. Advanced Data on Vital and Health Statistics, No. 92. Hyattsville, Md.: Public Health Service; DHHS Publication No. (PHS)83-1250.

USE OF SERVICES

Service use should be a reflection of population need. Medicare provides financial access to acute hospital care for the elderly, and increased financial access to physician care, particularly for hospital-based services but also for physician visits for the non-institutionalized population. Immediately following passage of Medicare there was an increase in the volume of hospital and physician services used by the elderly. This increase reflected in part an unmet need by those for whom there had been a problem in financial access prior to Medicare, as well as a continuing increase in need associated with an aging population. Most of the following data are for the decade 1971 to 1980, after the immediate impact of Medicare occurred.

Physician visits by the aged have declined slightly from 6.7 in 1964 to 6.6 in 1975 and 6.4 in 1980. The old do, however, have the highest visiting rates for internal medicine, general surgery, and family practice specialties.[20] Hospital discharge data indicate a continuing increase in hospitalizations for the aged between 1971 and 1980. There has been a decrease in length of stay for all ages including the elderly, as shown in Table 8. The rate of

TABLE 8   Hospital Discharges (in 1,000s), Average Length of Stay (Days), and Rate (per 1,000) for All Ages and the Aged for 1971, 1975, and 1980

	Year		
Age Group	1971	1975	1980
All ages			
Number of discharges	27,571	29,474	30,341
Average length of stay	8.5	8.0	7.6
Rate	136.2	141.0	139.3
65–74			
Number of discharges	2,613	2,969	3,805
Average length of stay	11.5	11.9	9.8
Rate	217.0	219.6	249.9
75+			
Number of discharges	1,952	2,349	2,808
Average length of stay	14.3	12.2	10.4
Rate	267.2	302.4	324.0

SOURCE: U.S. Department of Health and Human Services. National Center for Health Statistics, Public Health Service. Unpublished data from the National Health Interview Survey.

discharges per thousand remained constant overall but increased for the age group 65 to 74 by 15 percent and, for those 75 +, by 21 percent.

Of greater significance for the elderly population is the use of long-term care services. It is the amount of chronic disability and therefore the need for long-term care which most differentiates the old old population from younger aged. Among the elderly, it is the proportion of persons socially, mentally, and physically compromised among whom the need for long-term care is greatest. It is this population that is increasing most dramatically in number, whose financial resources are least, and therefore whose need for care is greatest, which poses the main challenge for the future.

The two major medical service elements of long-term care are nursing home and home care. Limited skilled nursing facility care is a Medicare benefit which until recently had to follow hospitalization. Intermediate care providing a combination of continuing nursing and personal care needs is a Medicaid but not a Medicare benefit. Under the stimulus of this increased financial access to intermediate and limited skilled nursing facility care, the number of nursing home beds increased 32 percent between 1969 and 1973–1974, another 21 percent in the ensuing three years to 1977, and a further 7 percent to 1980.[21] There has been a distinct tapering off in the rate of increase of nursing home beds as a result of certificate-of-need legislation and the increasing cost of capital for building.

The proportion of the population who are residents of nursing homes increases markedly with age—from 4.8 percent of the total population aged 65 and over to 23 percent of those 85 and over.[18] The 1977 National Nursing Home Survey demonstrated that length of stay increases substantially with age from a mean of 883 days for those 65 to 74, to 1,042 days for those 85 +, while the proportion of the nursing home population aged 85 and over rose from 28 to 35 percent between 1964 and 1977.[22,23] The low turnover, combined with high utilization by a steadily increasing population of the very old and a decline in the rate of increase to the stock of beds, will lead to a steady decrease in availability.

The rate of increase of nursing home utilization by the very old is exceeded only by the rate of increase in home health visits. The only national data available on home health visits over time is that provided by the Social Security Administration. Since

1972, Medicare has paid for home health visits for persons with defined medical need associated with an episode of illness. The number of home health visits under Medicare has been substantially increasing from 8.1 million visits in 1974 to 22.4 million in 1980. Persons served per 1,000 enrollees increased from 16.5 to 33.6 between 1974 and 1980, while visits per person served have increased from 20.6 to 23.4.[24] There is an increase in both the proportion of enrollees served and the intensity (frequency) of these visits. Table 9 shows that visits per 1,000 enrollees in a given year is a function of age, with nearly 600 percent more visits per 1,000 enrollees for those 85 + than for those aged 65 to 66. The intensity of visits per user is, however, the same for all age groups.[11]

Since the introduction of Medicare in 1966, there has been a change in the pattern of service use by the elderly. Except for physician visits there has been a greater increase in service use by the older aged. This has been particularly marked in long-term care services, that is, nursing home and home health agency use. Since these use patterns reflect the increasing morbidity of the old old, there is every reason to believe that the need for long-term care service will increase in the future as this population becomes more numerous. Changes in reimbursement policies will not affect the need for this care but might affect the demand and the ability to satisfy this need. Changes in service reimbursement must give consideration to the financial ability

TABLE 9　Use of Home Health Agency Services: Number of Visits (in 1,000s), Visits per User, and Visits per 1,000 Enrollees, 1980

Age	Number of Visits	Visits per User	Visits per 1,000 Enrollees
Total, all ages	22,428	23.4	788
65–66	1,084	22.4	303
67–68	1,324	22.4	397
69–70	1,515	22.9	497
71–72	1,665	22.9	595
73–74	1,789	23.1	727
75–79	4,758	23.4	989
80–84	4,261	23.2	1,383
85 +	4,226	23.7	1,753

SOURCE: U.S. Department of Health and Human Services. 1983. Health Care Financing Administration. Barrett, K. Personal communication and unpublished data.

of the affected population to pay for their care needs. Failure to do this will increase the financial burden upon the elderly for expensive home care and nursing home services. This inevitably will lead to a greater degree of medical indigency and greater public expenditures, if not under Medicare then under Medicaid.

MEDICAL CARE COSTS

While there has been an increase in the services consumed by the elderly, this increase in service use has been modest compared with the increase in medical care costs. From the perspective of public policy, increases in both public and private expenditure are important. Increases in public expenditure are visible; their magnitude has been great and has led to many recent Medicare changes. Some Medicare changes increase private expenditures for the elderly. Growth in these expenditures is less apparent than public expenditure but may ultimately be no less significant in determining public policy. It was, after all, the inability of the aged to meet health care costs that originally led to Medicare. If there are large segments of the elderly who are again unable to afford medical care, Medicare program changes are likely to be made.

With the initial passage of Medicare there was a marked shift in the pattern of payment for medical care expenses for the elderly, as shown in Table 10. Public expenditures for health care more than doubled from 30 to 61 percent between 1965 and 1970.[25] Percentage increases were particularly great for physician expenses, from 7 to 62 percent, and hospital expenses, from 49 to 89 percent. Federal expenditures for drugs and nursing homes increased less. In the period since, up to 1981, public expenditures for nursing homes and drugs have continued to rise. Medicaid now is responsible for 50 percent of nursing home and 18 percent of drug expenditures.

Meanwhile the proportion of private expenditure has increased slightly: for hospitals, from 11 to 14 percent, and for physicians, from 38 to 42 percent since 1970. Private expenditures changed very little between 1965 and 1970 in absolute terms, while public expenditures were increasing over fourfold as Medicare and Medicaid began to take effect. Since 1970 private health expenditures by the elderly have been increasing at a faster rate than public expenditures. Private expenditures for health care doubled by

TABLE 10   Aggregate Health Care Expenditures (in millions) for 65 + Population for Physicians' Services, Hospital Care, Drugs and Drug Sundries, and Nursing Home Care in 1965, 1970, 1976, and 1981; and Percent Expenditures From Public and Private Sources

Type of Expenditure	Total	Percent of All Ages	Private Funds	Percent of Total	Public Funds	Percent of Total
1965 total	$ 8,869	23.4	$ 6,213	70.0	$ 2,656	30.0
M.D.	1,737	20.5	1,617	93.1	120	6.9
Hospital	3,296	23.6	1,677	50.1	1,619	49.1
Drugs	1,148	20.0	1,030	89.7	118	10.3
Nursing home	1,825	88.1	1,187	65.0	638	35.0
1970 total	17,270	26.3	6,694	38.8	10,577	61.2
M.D.	3,030	21.1	1,166	38.5	1,864	61.5
Hospital	7,054	25.4	806	11.4	6,248	88.6
Drugs	1,732	20.6	1,524	88.0	208	12.0
Nursing home	4,144	88.6	2,255	54.4	1,889	45.6
1976 total	37,674	28.5	13,372	35.5	24,302	64.5
M.D.	6,505	23.5	2,746	42.2	3,759	58.8
Hospital	16,305	27.2	1,831	11.2	14,474	88.7
Drugs	2,716	21.2	2,263	83.3	453	16.7
Nursing home	9,395	82.0	4,693	50.0	4,702	50.0
1981 total	83,200	32.6	30,000	36.0	53,200	64.0
M.D.	15,600	28.5	6,600	42.3	9,000	57.7
Hospital	36,600	31.0	5,300	14.5	31,300	85.5
Drugs	5,100	23.8	4,200	82.3	900	17.6
Nursing home	19,400	80.1	9,600	49.5	9,800	50.5

SOURCE: Fischer, C. 1980. Differences by age groups in health care spending. Health Care Financing Report, 1:65–90; and unpublished 1981 data from Health Care Financing Administration, Bureau of Data Management and Strategy.

1976 and increased another two and a half times by 1981. From 1970 to 1981 private expenditures for health care increased from $6.7 billion to $30 billion. The major contributors to this cost increase are medical care inflation and increased need for services. Cost increases are greatest for hospital expenditures, which account for the largest portion of Medicare expenditures. Private expenditures consist of a combination of out-of-pocket expenditure and private insurance expenditures, including "medigap" insurance policies for those expenses not covered by Medicare. Expenditures go up with age in association with increased morbidity. This is reflected in Medicare expenditure data which show that total Medicare reimbursement per enrollee rises from $1,402 per person 65 to 69 to $2,485 for those 80 and above.[26] The same study showed 31 percent of those 80 + incurring high Medicare costs.

Just as older old persons incur more Medicare costs, they also have more out-of-pocket expenditures for medical expenses not covered by private insurance and Medicare. As shown in Table 3, there are sharp increases in death rates with successive age groups above 65 to 74. The rise in Medicare costs with age is due in part to medical expenses associated with the terminal episodes of disease. Lubitz and Prihoda demonstrated that 5 percent of Medicare enrollees in their last year of life accounted for 28 percent of total Medicare expenditures.[27] Over 90 percent of decedents used some Medicare-reimbursable service in the last year of life and 77 percent used services in the second-to-last year of life. Medicare spent 6.6 times as much on enrollees in their last year of life as on per capita expenditure for survivors, while for the second-to-last year of life expenditures were 2.3 times greater for those who had died than for those surviving.

Private medical expenditures are correlated with Medicare expenditures, increasing substantially with age. During a terminal illness expenditures may be enormous for acute care, as reflected in Medicare costs. Those unable to pay the rising medical care costs associated with old age become impoverished, and therefore eligible for Medicaid. Medicaid for the elderly will then pay for most medical care costs, though the extent varies from state to state. Personal care benefits are restricted, encouraging institutionalization for elderly with both health and personal care needs. If Medicaid patients are institutionalized in a nursing home, total costs are paid. This has encouraged the elderly to spend down their assets until they become eligible for Medicaid. The large number of institutionalized elderly in turn have caused the Medicaid program to become the major long-term care program as over one-third of Medicaid expenditures nationally are for nursing home care. To fully understand the problem of medical expenses for the elderly we must know more about the income and insurance status of the elderly.

INCOME AND THE AGED

One of the proud achievements of American society has been the reduction of poverty among the aged. When the Social Security Act was passed in the mid-1930s, most of the aged population was impoverished. Social Security Income Maintenance programs and, increasingly, accumulated wealth and private pensions decreased the proportions of the elderly in poverty to approximately 28 percent in 1965 and, following a substantial increase in Social Security payments in 1972, to 13.9 percent by 1978. By 1980 the figure increased slightly to 15.7 percent.[28] Social Security is the largest single source of income for most elderly, constituting an average of 37 percent of income for the total aged population.[29] The older the beneficiary, the more important is Social Security as a source of income, ranging from 28 percent at age 65 to 67 to 50 percent of income for those aged 80 +, as shown in Table 11. Though few are poor, the income of the elderly is not great, leaving little latitude for additional unexpected expenditures. The median personal income of the population aged 65 + in 1981 was $7,512, but this was unevenly distributed by age group, the median being $9,780 for those 65 to 67 and declining to $4,820 for those 80 +.

Medical care expenditures increased at a more rapid rate than the income of the elderly in the 1970s, but the proportion of personal income which paid for health expenditures has risen.

TABLE 11 Average Percentage Distribution of Money Income from Social Security and Other Sources for Age Groups 65 +, 1980

Age Group	Income Percent by Source	
	Social Security	Other Sources
Total 65 +	39	61
65–67	28	72
68–72	38	62
73–79	44	56
80 +	50	50

SOURCE: Department of Health and Human Services. 1983. Social Security Administration. Grad, S. Income of the Population 55 and Over 1980. Washington, D.C.: U.S. Government Printing Office; SSA Publication No. 13-11871.

Even before the effect of recent Medicare and Medicaid program changes, the percent of income spent on medical expenses by the elderly was 19.5 percent in 1981, rising to near the pre-Medicare level of 20.4 percent in 1965.[30] Recent Medicare program changes increase personal liability for medical care expenses substantially. For persons whose income is low, medical care expenditures loom large.

The one factor that separates the nonimpoverished elderly from out-of-pocket liability for medical care expenditures after Medicare is private health insurance. Having insurance is also age-related. According to the National Medical Care Expenditure Survey, in 1977, 70 percent of persons 65 to 74 had private insurance; this figure decreased to 60 percent for those 75 +.[31] Medigap insurance is often incomplete, covering only 6.6 percent of the aged's personal health expenditures, even though 36 percent of health expenditures by the elderly are private. According to the Health Insurance Association of America, in 1980 57 percent of persons 65 + had hospital insurance coverage, 42 percent had surgical coverage, and 40 percent had physician coverage.[32] Coverage for the long-term care expenses of nursing home and home care is uncommon and for drugs and laboratory tests for the elderly, rarer yet. Medigap policies mostly pay for Medicare coinsurance and deductibles. A typical annual premium cost from $300 to $400 per year in 1982. In recent years premium increases have been substantial, ranging up to 27 percent annually, sometimes with a decrease in benefits, making it even more difficult for the elderly to maintain even modest coverage.[30]

The very aged have least in the way of financial resources to pay for out-of-pocket expenditures or private health insurance. As a result, an increasing proportion of those well over 65 become impoverished, with the proportion of persons having both Medicare and Medicaid rising from 9 percent for those aged 65 to 69 to 13.5 percent of those 75 +, according to the National Medical Care Expenditure Survey of the noninstitutionalized population.[32] Currently it is estimated that 20 to 25 percent of the elderly are on Medicaid, including those in nursing homes.[33]

Although only 18 percent of persons on Medicaid are 65 +, medical payments for the elderly account for 39 percent of medical expenditures.[34] The disproportionate payment for the elderly is caused by nursing home expenditures, the single largest category of expenditure for state Medicaid programs. Despite state efforts to contain Medicaid nursing home reimbursement and to limit the number of nursing homes, the proportion of Medicaid expenditures devoted to nursing home care has continued at 35 percent, and Medicaid expenditures have continued to increase at an average of 17.7 percent per year through the 1970s, a rate in excess even of the increase in Medicare payments.[35]

A problem which became apparent during the rapid nursing home growth of the 1970s is that 25 to 40 percent of nursing home beds were filled by patients who could be maintained in the community. As a result of such findings and rising program costs, the states reduced the growth of nursing home beds and access to beds became more restricted. The inevitable result of the gradual aging of residents already in nursing homes, restrictions on admissions, and selective discharge of those most able to live in the community is that the population of patients remaining in nursing homes will become a more physically and mentally impaired group. This tendency was already apparent when the 1973–1974 and 1977 National Nursing Home surveys were compared for the activities of daily living status of the residents. Those not dependent in any activity of daily living decreased from 23.5 to 9.6 percent of residents while those dependent in all six assessed activities—bathing, dressing, toileting, mobility, continence, and eating—increased from 14.4 to 23.3 percent.[36]

With the reduced growth of nursing home beds and increase in the availability of home care, more old old will remain in the community. Indeed, even between 1973–1974 and 1977 the rate of those 85+ in nursing homes decreased from 254 to 216 per thousand.[23] With more old old in the community, the demand for community-based, long-term care services must increase. The Medicare figures on home care are the tip of the home care iceberg, as little personal care is provided under Medicare. Medicaid is more likely to pay for personal care, though most personal care is purchased by private payers. Most services consumed by disabled persons in the community are for personal care. The clients of the Triage Study in Connecticut used more companion and meal services than nursing and other physical care services. Homemaker and chore services were also widely used.[37]

THE MEDICARE AND MEDICAID DILEMMA

Medicare and Medicaid expenditures are distinctly different from those of other federal expenditures. Medical service expenditures are uncontrollable, as they result from legal entitlements to services. The costs of these uncontrollable services have increased at rates exceeding the growth of the national economy and other federal expenditures. Unsuccessful voluntary attempts to contain hospital costs under Medicare and continued growth of technology further frustrate the federal government. This frustration, combined with the election of President Ronald Reagan in 1980, who was committed to decreasing the size of the government and returning control to local and state officials, set the climate for Medicare and Medicaid reform.[38] The reforms were substantial and far-reaching, but they do not fundamentally reorganize the health care system. Some changes do provide new directions in the way health care is being financed, and these changes may lead to more fundamental reform.

Because of frustration over control of expenditures, the federal government is moving from a cost reimbursement to a price reimbursement system of payment. The most noteworthy of these changes is prospective reimbursement, which ultimately should diminish variations in the price of comparable services the federal government purchases, as well as contain the annual rate of increase in cost of similar services. The 1981 and 1982 changes in Medicare also initiated less widely known but similar types of limits on hospital ancillary services, renal dialysis, hospital physician reimbursement, home care, ambulatory surgery, and skilled nursing home care.

By moving to fixed reimbursement for newly available services, such as health maintenance organizations (HMOs) and hospice care, the federal government also initiated a formula for specified service within defined cost limits. Indeed the most far-reaching reform passed may be that of payment for hospice care. Under the hospice provisions the federal government will purchase a comprehensive package of services for a specific population, i.e., those terminally ill no longer receiving curative medical treatment. The services include the cost of institutional as well as home care, palliative drugs, medical counseling, and medical and social services, all as an integrated system of care, provided at a cost substantially less than would otherwise be expended in conventional medical and hospital care for similar patients.

Medicaid changes were no less profound. In addition to capping federal contributions under Medicaid, states were given greater program autonomy over which services to provide and how they should be provided. States may limit freedom-of-provider choice, develop new formulas for hospital reimbursement, and pay for community-based alternatives to institutional care. Each of these changes allows states to reimburse integrated health service systems; they allow negotiation between the state and providers regarding organization and price of care.

Despite these extensive program changes there continues to be a crisis in payment for medical care. Care is still an entitlement, though perhaps better regulated in price. Even with these far-reaching changes, spending for Medicare and Medicaid programs is likely to be $100 billion in 1985. The Medicare Hospital Insurance Trust Fund will not remain solvent. As projected by the Congressional Budget Office, by the year 1988 the Hospital Insurance Fund will be in deficit.[26] The substantial Medicare changes of the last two years have not resolved the short-term crisis in Medicare funding, nor is the desirability of expanding coverage fulfilled. The Medicare Advisory Panel is recommending an increase in both program charges and benefits. Increased income would come from substantially higher beneficiary contributions. This would pay for additional days of care and limit out-of-pocket expenditures for an episode of illness. The recommendations leave unresolved the problem of how those who most need the benefit, the severely ill and the old old, would afford increased premiums and additional out-of-pocket costs for initial days of hospitalization.[39]

THE MEDICAL CARE DILEMMA

The financial problem is not the only one facing the health care delivery system in relation to the old and the aged. Medicare successfully reduced the financial liability of the elderly for acute care but contributed to the development of new problems, only a portion of which relate to medical care costs. Once a patient requires long-term care, he requires services with which physicians responsible for acute care are unfamiliar.

Physicians caring for those needing long-term care, particularly the old old, are treating patients with multiple medical, economic, and social needs. The understanding of their medical need is continually changing and becoming more complicated. The scientific base underlying the physiology of the normal aged is steadily being developed. There are many normal, age-related biochemical and physiologic changes that affect physical, pharmacologic, metabolic, and recuperative functions of the aged. These underlying normal physiologic changes are further complicated by an infinite combination of diseases in patients and an increasing number of therapeutic and diagnostic procedures. Few physicians can keep up with this new knowledge or incorporate it into practice.

Long-term care patients need services with which most physicians are not only unfamiliar but over which they have little control. The physician has little responsibility for patient care in nursing homes and is discouraged from frequent attendance by low reimbursement rates for visits and disallowances for too-frequent visits. Patients in nursing homes, if given up by their physicians as commonly occurs with Medicaid patients, have major problems in communicating their care needs when referred for acute care to a hospital and when they return to the nursing home.

As with nursing home care, reimbursement policies discourage home care. Few physicians are trained in home care or understand differences in levels of home care, types of home care services, or personal care. Home care agencies have difficulty communicating with private physicians. Yet these services need to be prescribed by physicians in order for the patient to secure third party reimbursement. Patients requiring personal care by homemakers or private agencies are therefore even further removed from the care of physicians than those in nursing homes.

The recognition of these problems has led to discussion of the need for geriatric specialists in care of the frail elderly: a physician who can lead patients and families through the maze of medical and social services and help them in adjusting to the ever-changing demands of progressive disease processes and decreasing physiologic and social functioning. The lack of coordination of the diverse and changing needs of patients requiring long-term care makes effective care provision difficult. Such difficulty may contribute to physical deterioration, which in turn leads to the need for high-cost episodes of acute hospital care. Many old old long-term care patients must make complex decisions about sources of medical and personal care when they are ill, vulnerable, and confused. Family, often removed from continual contact with the patient, are no more knowledgeable about the subtleties of long-term care services. Though they are better able to become informed, they may be concerned about their own liability for providing or paying for needed personal care. They may feel conflict from knowledge that more intensive, no-cost service provision at home or in a nursing home is available if the older person becomes impoverished and receives Medicaid.

A PROPOSAL

Instead of concern for acute medical care, the most predictable concern of the long-lived is the risk of need for long-term care and its disastrous social and financial consequences. Few old old have the financial resources to pay for such care and its consequences, and insurance does not cover it. Failure to provide effective long-term care exacerbates the need for expensive reimbursable acute care. Many of those surviving long enough will eventually become impoverished by the cost of medical care and become public wards in their last years. All those 85 + will eventually be terminal; they all have high risk of an expensive one-to-two years of service use. That many of these vulnerable long-lived people will become paupers makes no sense in human terms nor, often, in medical terms. Our medical payment mechanism should provide what is needed for these people, not according to their financial status but on the basis of medical need.

Many aged requiring long-term care become confused as to their priority needs, divided as these needs are among many different medical and nonmedical providers. Each provider has different incentives for providing care and varying techniques for handling problems. Mechanisms for obtaining interprofessional communication with regard to patient needs hardly exist; information and communication are not reimbursable. Rarely is care managed through multidisciplinary teams of providers brought together for diagnosis and management of medically and socially compromised patients. At the same time there are few areas where care needs are so broad and interrelated. Many needs can be satisfied by minimally trained but well-intentioned people. Given a coordinating mechanism, substitution of high-skilled by low-skilled persons or volunteers can be accomplished. What is lacking is a mechanism to encourage social, nursing, and medical professionals to cooperate for the best needs of the patient at an acceptable and predictable price. To permit the greatest benefit in care and cost savings, a closer amalgamation of long-term with acute care is needed. The inappropriateness of paying for expensive physician-intensive care and failure to encourage less intensive nursing and personal care is becoming less tolerable with the increasing numbers of old old. The financial needs of the aged, the economic constraints of society, and the professional need to provide more coordinated care should all serve as an impetus for change. The passage of hospice legislation offers a precedent under Medicare for payment of integrated services. The hospice benefit allows for a greater range and for more substitutability in filling the needs of patients requiring social, nursing, and medical care than exists under the Medicare reimbursement system for acute care. The Medicaid experiences of many states in developing alternative methods of community and medical care will provide further experience in developing a coordinated system for both acute and long-term care needs.

For the elderly, the major health expenditure is for acute hospital care. Programs which include these services as part of a service benefit could provide experience which might be applied in developing a coordinated acute, long-term, and community care package. Such a package would permit more appropriate and integrated use of medical, social, and community support services. Medicare and Medicaid experience with the purchase of price-defined service packages would assure both service coordination and cost containment.

We should recognize the old old as being medically and socially distinct and provide them with a total care benefit as a right, whether it is in the acute hospital for terminal illness, in an intermediate care facility, or in the home. Such an approach would ensure that the elderly did not suffer the indignity of impoverishment by health care costs, would demonstrate the will of society to care for its frailest members, and could provide a direction for the development of the overall health care system.

SUMMARY

Following the introduction of Medicare and Medicaid in 1966, both federal and state governments were faced with escalating program costs and crises in acute and long-term medical care. This led to measures that have decreased services, withdrawn eligibility, or shifted a higher burden of costs to the consumer.

At the same time, those for whom the programs were introduced are becoming "older" as mortality rates have declined. There is now a significant and growing proportion of the population aged 85 and over. It is this group of frail "old old" who have multiple morbidity combined with a complex of social needs. They also have low and declining incomes and are least able to meet health care costs.

The complex needs of this group conflict with the ability of our fragmented and uncoordinated health and social system to provide appropriate care. No one professional group can assess, organize, and provide for their needs. Meeting these needs is costly. Government is unlikely to provide unrestrained financial access to additional services. Provision of multiple services for the old old should be more efficiently coordinated across the range of both acute and long-term care requirements.

Medicare itself could be the precedent for introducing another age-related entitlement for those reaching 85. This precedent, combined with the recent passage of provider reimbursement on a price-for-service basis, as well as hospice legislation, offers a framework for meeting service needs.

Provision of integrated medical and social support services within acceptable price limits to those 85 + would fulfill society's obligation to the oldest, frailest, and most needy, without imposing on them the indignity of impoverishment.

ACKNOWLEDGMENTS

The author wishes to acknowledge with appreciation Margaret Haske for her essential assistance in data collection for this manuscript and the assistance of Irene McDonald in its final preparation.

NOTES

1. U.S. Department of Commerce. 1981. Bureau of the Census. Decennial Census of the Population 1900–1980. Washington, D.C.: U.S. Government Printing Office.

2. U.S. Department of Commerce. 1983. Bureau of the Census. Projections of the Population of the United States: 1982–2050 (Advance Report). Current Population Reports, Series P-25, No. 922. Washington, D.C.: U.S. Government Printing Office.

3. U.S. Department of Commerce. 1983. Bureau of the Census. Passel, J. Personal communication.

4. U.S. Department of Health and Human Services. 1982. National Center for Health Statistics, Public Health Service. Annual Summary of Births, Deaths, Marriages, and Divorces: United States, 1981. Monthly Vital Statistics Report, Vol. 30, No. 13. Hyattsville, Md.: Public Health Service; DHHS Publication No. (PHS)83-1120.

5. Crimmins, E. 1983. Recent and Prospective Trends in Old Age Mortality. Paper presented at the Annual Meeting of the American Association for the Advancement of Science, Detroit.

6. Brody, J., and D. B. Brock. Epidemiologic Characteristics of the United States Elderly Population in the Twentieth Century. Draft paper, National Institute on Aging, Bethesda, Md.

7. U.S. Department of Health and Human Services. 1982. National Center for Health Statistics, Public Health Service. Final Mortality Statistics, 1979. Monthly Vital Statistics Advance Report, Supplement. Hyattsville, Md.: Public Health Service; DHHS Publication No. (PHS)82-1230.

8. Baum, H. M., and M. Goldstein. 1982. Cerebrovascular disease type specific mortality: 1968–1977. Stroke 13:6.

9. Levy, R. I., and G. W. Ward. 1979. Hypertension control: A succeeding national effort. Journal of the American Medical Association 241:2546.

10. U.S. Department of Health and Human Services. 1981. Health—United States: 1981. Washington, D.C.: U.S. Government Printing Office; DHEW Publication No. (PHS)82-1232.

11. U.S. Department of Health and Human Services. 1977. National Center for Health Statistics, Public Health Service. Unpublished data from the National Health Interview Survey.

12. U.S. Department of Health and Human Services. 1983. National Center for Health Statistics, Public Health Service. Feller, B. A. Americans Needing Help to Function at Home. Advance Data From Vital and Health Statistics, No. 92. Hyattsville, Md.: Public Health Service; DHHS Publication No. (PHS)83-1250.

13. Mortimer, J. A., L. M. Schuman, and L. R. French. 1981. Epidemiology of dementing illness. Pp. 3–23 in Mortimer, J. A., and L. M. Schuman, eds. The Epidemiology of Dementia. New York: Oxford University Press.

14. Kramer, M. The rising pandemic of mental disorders and associated chronic diseases and disabilities. In Epidemiologic Research as Basis for the Organization of Extramural Psychiatry. Acta Psychiatrica Scandinavia, Suppl. 285, Vol. 62.

15. Brody, J. A., and L. R. White. 1982. The epidemiology of mental disorders: Results from the Epidemiologic Catchment Area Study (ECA). Psychopharmacology Bulletin, Vol. 18, July.

16. Sluss, T. K., E. M. Gruenberg, and M. Kramer. 1981. The use of longitudinal studies in the investigation of risk factors for senile dementia—Alzheimer type. Pp. 132–154 in Mortimer, J. A., and L. M. Schuman, eds. The Epidemiology of Dementia. New York: Oxford University Press.

17. Blazer, D. 1985. Depressive Illness in Late Life. In this volume.

18. U.S. Department of Health and Human Services. 1979. National Center for Health Statistics, Public Health Service. National Nursing Home Survey: 1977, Summary for the United States. National Health Survey, Series 13, No. 43. Washington, D.C.: U.S. Government Printing Office; DHEW Publication No. (PHS)79-1794.

19. Katzman, R. 1985. Age and Age-Dependent Disease: Cognition and Dementia. In this volume.

20. U.S. Department of Health and Human Services. 1982. Health—United States: 1982. Hyattsville, Md.: Public Health Service; DHHS Publication No. (PHS)83-1232.

21. U.S. Department of Health and Human Services. 1977. Health—United States: 1976–1977. Washington, D.C.: Government Printing Office; DHEW Publication No. (HRA)77-1232.

22. U.S. Department of Health and Human Services. 1973. National Center for Health Statistics, Public Health Service. Characteristics of Residents in Nursing and Personal Care Homes: United States, June–August, 1969. National Health Survey, Series 12, No. 19. Washington, D.C.: U.S. Government Printing Office; DHEW Publication No. (HSM)73-1704.

23. U.S. Department of Health and Human Services. 1981. National Center for Health Statistics, Public Health Service. Characteristics of Nursing Home Residents: National Nursing Home Survey, United States, May–December, 1977. National Health Survey, Series 13, No. 51. Washington, D.C.: U.S. Government Printing Office; DHEW Publication No. (PHS)81-1712.

24. U.S. Department of Health and Human Services. 1983. Health Care Financing Administration. Barrett, K. personal communication. Unpublished data.

25. C. Fischer. 1980. Differences by age groups in health care spending. Health Care Financing Report, 1:65-90.

26. Congressional Budget Office. 1983. Changing the Structure of Medicare Benefits: Issues and Options. Washington, D.C.: U.S. Government Printing Office.

27. U.S. Department of Health and Human Services. 1984. Health—United States, 1983. Lubitz, J., and R. Prihoda. Use and Costs of Medicare Services in the Last Years of Life. Washington, D.C.: U.S. Government Printing Office; DHHS Publication No. (PHS)84-1232.

28. Retirement Income. 1983. Developments in Aging, 1982, Vol. 1; Part I; A Report of the Senate Special Committee on Aging. Washington, D.C.: U.S. Government Printing Office, 1983.

29. C. Taeuber. 1983. America in Transition: An Aging Society. Developments in Aging, 1982, 1:1-41; A Report of the Senate Special Committee on Aging. Washington, D.C.: U.S. Government Printing Office.

30. Health Care Expenditures for the Elderly: How Much Protection Does Medicare Provide? 1982. Information paper prepared by the staff of the Special Committee on Aging, United States Senate, Washington, D.C.: U.S. Government Printing Office.

31. U.S. Department of Health and Human Services. National Center for Health Services Research. National Medical Care Expenditure Survey, 1977. Unpublished data.

32. Ward, R., ed. 1982. Source Book of Health Insurance Data: 1981–1982. Washington, D.C.: Health Insurance Association of America.

33. Crisis in Health Care. 1983. Briefing paper prepared by the staff of the Subcommittee on Health and Long-Term Care, House Select Committee on Aging.

34. Muse, A., and A. Sawyer. 1982. The Medicare and Medicaid Data Book. Washington, D.C.: U.S. Government Printing Office; HCFA Publication No. 03128.

35. Etheridge, L., J. Merrill, and K. Tyson. 1983. The President's 1984 Budget: An Analysis. Washington, D.C.: Georgetown University Center for Health Policy Studies.

36. Government Accounting Office. 1982. Preliminary Findings on Patient Characteristics and State Medicaid Expenditures for Nursing Home Care. Washington, D.C.: U.S. Government Printing Office; GAO Report IPE-82-4.

37. Hicks, B., and J. L. Quinn. 1979. Triage: Coordinated Delivery of Services to the Elderly. Grant No. HSO 2563, National Center for Health Services Research, Office of Assistant Secretary of Health, U.S. Department of Health and Human Services, Washington, D.C.

38. Etheridge, L. 1983. Reagan, Congress, and Health Spending. Health Affairs, Spring.

39. Rich, S. 1983. Medicare panel votes cost benefit increase. Washington Post, June 22.

Active Life Expectancy: Societal Implications

Sidney Katz,* David S. Greer, John C. Beck,
Laurence G. Branch, and William D. Spector

In a 1983 paper, we demonstrated the use of life table techniques to describe the health of people in a large area—in terms of function.[1] The population was the noninstitutional elderly in Massachusetts in 1974, and level of health was described in terms of the degree of independence or dependence in activities of daily living (ADL), measured by a modified form of the Index of ADL.[2,3] Information about the population's functional health experience was summarized in the form of Active Life Expectancy tables, according to methods traditionally used to summarize life expectancy for large populations.[4]

In the study described above, we observed that the active life expectancy of the noninstitutional elderly of Massachusetts decreased with age from 10 years for people entering the age category of 65 to 70 years to 2.9 years for those 85 and older (Table 1).[1] Active life expectancy (ALE) was longer for the nonpoor than the poor of every age group, ranging from 2.4 additional years for the nonpoor who were 65 to 70 years old to 0.6 additional year for those 85 and older. Overall, no remarkable sex difference in ALE together with a longer life expectancy of women, resulted

*Associate Dean of Medicine, Director, Southeastern New England Long Term Care Gerontology Center, Brown University, Providence, Rhode Island. Paper was prepared for the Institute of Medicine and was supported in part by the Administration on Aging (Older Americans Act, Title IV-E, 90 AT-2164).

TABLE 1 Active Life Expectancy (Remaining Years
of Independent Activities of Daily Living),
Noninstitutional Elderly, Massachusetts, 1974[a]

Age	Type of Person	Active Life Expectancy
65–70	All	10.0
	Nonpoor	10.5
	Poor	8.1
70–75	All	8.1
	Nonpoor	8.3
	Poor	6.8
75–80	All	6.8
	Nonpoor	6.9
	Poor	6.1
80–85	All	4.7
	Nonpoor	4.8
	Poor	4.4
85+	All	2.9
	Nonpoor	3.1
	Poor	2.5

[a]Data are from the first and second waves of the Massachusetts
Health Care Panel Study (ref. 1).

in a longer average duration of expected dependency for women
than for men in all age groups.

The purpose of the present paper is to discuss the societal implications of ALE in the context of the changing age distribution
of our population. In the next section, we address briefly the
genesis and nature of the ALE concept and the approach used to
develop information about ALE. We then discuss its implications.

BACKGROUND

Information about life expectancy has served many purposes.
Among these, it has focused attention on differences in the health
of large populations and subgroups, leading to targeted policies
aimed at improving health. Thus, for example, the observed high
infant mortality in developing countries has contributed to efforts
to address problems of infectious disease and nutrition in those
countries.[5,6] Increased mortality associated with carcinogens in
the workplace and excess exposure to radioactivity have led to
protective legislation and regulation.[7] Projections in life expec-

tancy have helped planners to estimate years of life lost and to delineate health problems in subgroups of the population or in particular geographic areas.[8,9] Projections of life expectancy have also been used as actuarial information on which to base cost estimates for insurance.[10]

Mortality statistics revealed the changing nature of major diseases in the United States from infectious diseases in the nineteenth century to chronic diseases in the mid-twentieth century.[6,11] More recently, mortality due to cardiovascular disease has decreased in the United States, a decline possibly related to efforts in health promotion and disease prevention, i.e., less smoking, more exercising, better diet habits, and improved control of hypertension.[11–13] Mortality statistics in terms of life expectancy have also revealed differences related to age, sex, and economic status. In addition to usefulness in policy-making and planning, this information has provided direction to investigators who seek to explain the causes of decreased life expectancy and who seek to find ways of improving health.

Despite the continuing usefulness of mortality and life expectancy as measures of the health of a population, use of death as an endpoint of health has certain limitations. As populations approach the biological limits of the natural life span, the technologies for treating diseases have a diminishing effect on life expectancy, and increases in life expectancy become harder to attain.[14,15] The aging population has more chronic conditions and more disability. There is a related increase in expenditures for health care with age, and the last year of life is now the most costly year in terms of care. By definition, services in the last year of life do not buy a longer life, and one must ask whether the costly services buy a better life. Death, as the endpoint, measures the former but not the latter. In the absence of suitable options for measuring health and in the context of our aging society, we believe that the exclusive reporting of health in terms of mortality and life expectancy focuses disproportionately, and often inappropriately, on achieving a longer life rather than on achieving life of a better quality. Policy-makers, planners, providers, and the general public need other information in order to allocate resources in a balanced way between efforts to produce a long life and a life of high quality.

We recognize that quality is a multidimensional concept and varies with the viewpoint of the observer.[16] For example, there are physical, psychological, social, and economic interpretations of quality. Quality also encompasses both objective and subjective considerations. Thus, the operational definitions of quality must be specified clearly in order to represent accurately the viewpoint of quality that is intended. With regard to aging and the increased likelihood of both dysfunction and long-term care, functional well-being is widely recognized as among the most important considerations in the quality of life.

Since we measured active life expectancy in terms of basic ADL functions, a brief description is in order of the history of functional assessment in populations and of the background of the ADL concept within that historical context. In the late 1800s and the early 1900s, in Europe and in the United States, information about functional status was obtained in health interview surveys.[17,18] These surveys were intended to obtain data about prevalent morbidity in large populations. Information was reported in terms of days of sickness per person or per 1,000 persons and in terms of the number of persons who were sick and unable to work on the day of the interview. This information represented an early example of the application of contemporary concepts of disability or dysfunction in the measurement of health status. These measures were later refined by the introduction of questions about duration—for example, about sickness during the preceding year—and about information on the seasonal duration of illness.[17,19,20] In addition, a service-related interest was represented by the appearance of use:need ratios in survey reports, e.g., person-days of hospitalization per 100 days of disability.[21] The introduction of information about restricted activities, mobility, and activities of daily living as categories of function occurred in the 1940s and 1950s. [18,22–24] More recently, there has been an increased behavioral orientation in information about dysfunction.[24–26]

As the content of health surveys broadened, methods of measurement were refined. For example, periodic interviewing at 2-week intervals was introduced as a strategy to solve problems of recall.[27–31] Diary-keeping in the Eastern Health District Study served the same purpose.[20,32–36] That study also used a hierarchically ordered classification of dysfunction and intensity of services as a means of evaluating severity of illness.

In recognition of the increasing importance of chronic diseases and long-term care, the Commission on Chronic Illness was established in 1949 with a mandate to study the chronic illness problem in the United States. The Commission extended methodologic studies in the area of sampling, in classifying severity of illness, in multiphasic screening, and in follow-up techniques.[22,37-39] The use:need ratio introduced by the Canadian Sickness Survey provided a new method of measuring the distribution of need for care.[21] In the San Jose Survey of 1957, ways of collecting data from populations chosen by objective sampling techniques were studied, as well as ways of linking data obtained from medical records to data collected by other methods such as interviewing, diary-keeping, and continuing observations of panels.[40] The California Health Survey of 1954–1955 contributed information about respondent bias, response variability, and the measurement of disability.[40] Importantly, the National Center for Health Statistics, established in 1956, made significant contributions to defining and measuring such elements of information as chronic conditions, restricted activities, mobility, activity limitations, and impairments.[41-42] The Health Survey of Finland in the 1960s introduced measurement of perceived morbidity as another basis for assessing need.[26]

In addition to methodologic refinements from survey research on health status, contributions were made by research that focused particularly on methods of measurement and classification. For example, Fanshel and Bush[43] and Lerner[44] conceived of health status as a continuum of a broad spectrum of functions and dysfunctions. Fanshel and Bush,[43] Miller,[45] and Sullivan[46] studied preference weights in the quantification of health status. Jones, McNitt, and McKnight[47] developed a classification system that included the most important current elements of measures of health status in long-term care.

As measures of health evolved during the early 1950s, the Commission on Chronic Illness expressed the need for a classification of activities of daily living. Among several investigators who responded to this need, Katz and co-workers developed and used an Index of ADL whose grades reflect degree of disability. Each grade summarizes the profile of an individual's overall level of disability as measured in six basic functions: bathing, dressing, toileting, transfer, continence, and feeding.[2] Parallels between the order of these functions and the pattern of child growth and development suggest that the Index is based on essential biological functions. The hierarchical nature of the Index of ADL allows one to rank people in an ordered manner, to compare individuals or groups, and to detect changes over time.

In early studies the Index of ADL was shown to be reliable, and its wide range of usefulness has been demonstrated repeatedly since that time.[2,48] The Index was used to produce predictive information about specific chronic diseases. It also contributed to the epidemiologic and experimental study of chronic illnesses and aging. For example, 10-year follow-up studies of patients with fracture of the hip and stroke revealed that the likelihood of recovery decreased over time in the presence of sophisticated rehabilitation services.[49,50] The likelihood of recovery of function virtually disappeared 18 to 24 months after the onset of disability, if such function had not returned by that time. This information had implications for the definition of criteria with regard to the duration, delivery, and financing of technology-rich rehabilitation services.

In a controlled study of comprehensive outpatient care of rheumatoid arthritis patients, coordinated care was provided by a team of physicians, nurses, and social workers.[51] It was found that coordinated outpatient treatment, when compared to the usual form of care, was beneficial in terms of clinical manifestations of the disease. More improvements and fewer deteriorations in economic dependence were also evident, as well as fewer regressions in daily living activities.

The multidisciplinary studies of aging and chronic illness referred to above were followed by two major experimental studies. The first of these studies, conducted in Cleveland, Ohio, was the Continued Care Study.[52] The second study, conducted in Michigan, was the Chronic Disease Module Study.[53]

In the Continued Care Study, patients 50 years and older discharged home from a chronic disease rehabilitation hospital were randomly assigned to a treatment or to a control group.[52] The treatment consisted of regular visits to the patient's home by a public health nurse, working with the patient's physician and community resources. Follow-up observations were made through home visits over a 2-year period following each patient's discharge. It was found that relatively young (50 to 64 years), less disabled, and less severely ill persons were more likely to benefit in physical and mental function after receiving long-term visiting nurse services than were similar people in a control group who did not receive such services. Admissions to nursing homes were also delayed among people who received visiting nurse services. In contrast, the presence of visiting nurse services was associated with an increased use of hospitals and professionals among the oldest, very disabled, and most severely ill people when compared to similar persons in a control group. Despite an increased use of services, the high-risk group (older, very disabled, and severely ill) did not benefit in physical and mental function in the presence of the visiting nurse program.

The Chronic Disease Module Study, a 5-year experimental project, was a logical extension of the previous study.[53] In this study, a less costly service was provided: a program of continuing home visits by health assistants who worked with a small team consisting of a physician and a nurse or social worker. The acceptance, outcome, and costs of this service were evaluated. Patients in selected ambulatory care facilities or those who were about to be discharged from acute care hospitals in five Michigan communities were randomly assigned to treatment or control groups. The study results showed that relatively young, less disabled, and less severely ill people experienced higher levels of satisfaction and morale after receiving home services by a health assistant than did similar people in a control group who did not receive such services. Avoidance of functional deterioration was not demonstrated as an effect of home care by health assistants.

On the basis of the foregoing experience with longitudinal studies of disabled people, it was concluded that service goals shift over time after the onset of disability. Use of technology-rich or intensive medical and rehabilitative services to effect improvement is appropriate for about a year, at the most 2 years after onset. Thereafter, service goals are more appropriately defined as maintenance of function, support of social needs, and access to more sophisticated services at times of increased need. This implies that long-term services for people with less potential for improvement should be organized with more emphasis on planning, teaching, monitoring, support, and coordination than on intensive treatment modalities. An issue to be resolved in this regard is the way of introducing appropriate changes in the balance between supportive services and technology-rich services over time.

Widespread use of ADL measures was documented in a recent report of 14 surveys which provided information about the prevalence of chronic conditions and need for services, plus 22 studies of changes in health status.[18] For example, the Index of ADL was used in the U.S. National Nursing Home Survey to describe the 1,303,100 residents of the nation's 18,900 nursing homes in 1977.[54] Other examples included a longitudinal study of nursing home residents; an experimental study of day care and homemaker services in six demonstration sites across the country; and the Panel Study, which served as the source of the ALE data reported here.[3,55,56]

There is broadly based agreement that basic ADL functions are relevant to the aging process and to long-term care. Most classification systems used to describe the functional health of the aged incorporate the six functions of the Index of ADL. For example, the well-documented usefulness of the Index has led to its inclusion in two contemporary systems for the classification of long-term care patients. One is the *Patient Classification for Long-Term Care: User's Manual.*[47] The second system is the *Long-Term Health Care: Minimum Data Set*, developed under the sponsorship of the National Center for Health Statistics.[57]

Experiences such as these provide guiding principles about (a) the goals that are likely to be achieved by different categories of service programs, and (b) the types of people who are likely to respond to each form of service. The experiences also demonstrate the usefulness and validity of information systems that use ADL to assess the needs of clients or patients and their responses to care.

IMPLICATIONS

Information about active life expectancy should play an important part in rationalizing planning and reimbursement for nursing home care. Nursing home expenditures in the United States in 1977 were $12.8 billion, representing 12 percent of public expenditures for all of personal health care.[58] Of the $12.8 billion, $7.3 billion or 57 percent was from the federal government. Medicaid paid $6.3 billion (one-third of the Medicaid budget), while Medicare, the Veterans Administration, state, and local resources accounted for the remaining $1.2 billion. Private funding accounted for almost one-half (45.4 percent) of all nursing home expenditures, primarily paid out-of-pocket by residents and their families. Although the public–private split for nursing homes was about the same as for hospitals, third party expenditures accounted for only 1.6 percent of private expenditures, while the corresponding percentage was 33.8 percent for hospitals.[58]

Of importance to public policy and planning is the fact that nursing home expenditures have continued to increase at a significant rate, as reflected by increases of about 17.4 percent per year between 1976 and 1979. The pressures will be further magnified by projected increases in the nursing home population. Based on projections of population growth and available age-specific nursing home admission rates, it has been estimated that there will be a 54 percent increase in the nursing home population by the year 2000 and a 132 percent increase by the year 2030.[58] Thus, the present situation is one of (a) increasing nursing home expenditures with increasing numbers of people in nursing homes, (b) decreasing public funding, (c) increasing private funding in the absence of significant third party response, and (d) greater cost to the nursing home resident and family.

With regard to long-term care insurance, an important barrier to public and private initiatives has been the perception that actuarial data for rational cost estimates have not been available. As a result, private insurers have not assumed responsibility for long-term care to the degree that they have for hospital care, and Medicaid has been burdened by costs that have not been based on adequate planning. The absence of a sound actuarial base has also limited policy-making with regard to resource development and its allocation. Based on the proposed technique for producing Active Life Expectancy tables, expectancy information can now be developed for the various degrees of dysfunction that lead to entry into the main parts of the long-term care system. For example, incontinence and immobility are important dysfunctions that lead to nursing home admission, while dysfunction of lesser degrees leads to informal or formal care at home. Since different goals have different endpoints, expectancy estimates can be developed for each component of the long-term care system.

Most long-term care agents (home care programs, chronic disease hospitals, nursing homes, etc.) currently evaluate their activities in terms of information about the structural characteristics of their separate programs, types of clients or patients served, utilization counts, and costs of services. In instances where changes are described in the well-being of clients or patients, standard bases for comparison are not available. In the absence of population norms, cost-effectiveness is either not evaluated or tends to be evaluated in terms of measures that are biased toward the norms of the reporting agency or institution. As a consequence, many separate services and service imperatives prevail, rather than systems of integrated community services. Separateness and inadequately stable criteria for admission and discharge make it almost impossible to identify duplication and fragmentation.

The availability of a measure of active life expectancy provides a new tool for addressing some important systems issues in long-term care. Subgroup-specific information about active life expectancy would provide normative information against which to examine the relative effects of services and, ultimately, their cost-effectiveness. Information about cost-effectiveness would provide a way of evaluating criteria for service entry and discharge. In the context of the existing range of services and the needs of the elderly population in a given community, the process of examining cost-effectiveness would also contribute to the evaluation of duplication and fragmentation. The net result would be stimulation and development of more rational systems of long-term care.

Comparison of expectancy estimates among subgroups of the population would help to identify needy groups. Priorities could then be established, and assistance could be targeted. For example, the shorter active life expectancy of the poor in Massachusetts should be addressed, as well as the shorter active life expectancy of the very old who are most likely to be ill, to have lost their informal supports, and to enter nursing homes. Additional subgroup comparisons are needed with regard to education, occupation, living arrangements, and disease status. We know, for example, that elderly people with less education are more likely to be poor. Thus, it is likely that education, income, and active life expectancy are interrelated. Data about the interrelationship would provide a better basis on which to plan for future services than is now possible. Similarly, disease-specific rates of active life expectancy would help us make better policy decisions about both the direction and rate of development of service technologies for specific diseases.

Currently, efforts in prevention deal mostly with primary and secondary prevention, i.e., averting diseases, injuries, or defects and early detection of disease. Much less attention is focused on tertiary prevention, that is, efforts to improve residual function, to prevent the progression of disability, and to improve the quality of life. The balance in the focus of health policies between these types of prevention should be changed toward a greater emphasis on tertiary prevention in view of the aging of the population, the increasing importance of chronic diseases, and the high cost of long-term care. We believe that necessary changes in current health policies are hampered by the absence of sound information about the functional determinants of health and the functional outcomes of services, since that is the domain of tertiary prevention. Information about active life expectancy, in objective terms, would bring the issue of tertiary prevention to the attention of the public, providers, and policy-makers. Issues of quality of life could then be addressed, and appropriate changes in health policy would become possible. Information about disease and death would not be the overriding stimulus for health policy. Health policy could increasingly take into account the uniqueness of problems of and services for the elderly. For example, the unique importance of function to the well-being of the elderly could be reflected in new coordinated approaches to the allocation of social and health resources.

For research, the focus on active life expectancy and functional health brings new challenges. Research priorities, which currently reflect a primary emphasis on elucidating the causes and mechanisms of disease, should be modified to include at least equal emphasis on the causes and mechanisms of dysfunction. Comparative information that we developed about active life expectancy in Massachusetts indicated that the poor were at high risk of having shorter active life expectancies than the nonpoor. What biological, psychological, and socioeconomic factors explain this risk? When the risk factors are clarified, strategies to improve the outcome can be developed and tested. A challenging set of both basic and applied questions for research become apparent.

Another example of research implications of the active life expectancy study in Massachusetts emerges from the observation that women and men older than 70 years did not differ noticeably with regard to active life expectancy. Since women live longer than men, on the average, the absence of a difference in active life expectancy indicates that dependent women survive longer than dependent men. Do women tolerate the stresses of dependency better than men, and, if so, what biological, psychological, and socioeconomic factors explain this observation? What strategies can be developed and tested to increase the active life expectancy of both men and women? What can be learned from an understanding of the basic mechanisms of stress tolerance that can be used to improve the quality of life?

An important series of questions derives from previous knowledge about the sequence of loss and return of ADL functions among the elderly. For example, recovery of individual ADL functions in certain disabled patients has been shown to parallel the normal order of development of the same functions in young children, implying that there may be a biological order to the gain and loss of ADL functions in the elderly. Thus, it appears that prevention or delay of dependence in bathing and dressing could delay disability of greater severity. As a related assumption, institutionalization could be delayed or prevented by early efforts designed to control the many instances of incontinence which are modifiable. Basic and applied research in these areas could have an important influence on the quality of life and on policy directions.

SUMMARY

The concept of active life expectancy expands the available kinds of measures of health in large populations, adding a measure of functional health to the currently used measure of death. Implementation of the ALE concept was demonstrated in a previously reported study of the noninstitutional elderly population of Massachusetts in 1974. In that study, functional health expectancy was summarized with the aid of life table methodology, using a measure of activities of daily living as the endpoint instead of death. Based on the experience with the Massachusetts study, this paper has addressed the societal implications of the ALE approach in the context of the aging population of the United States.

The authors believe that appropriately detailed information about ALE would contribute to an improved actuarial base for long-term care insurance. Such information would also provide normative information about the functional health of populations that would serve as standards for comparison and would be useful in evaluating the relative effects of alternative services. Information about ALE would help to identify groups in need and would contribute to the development of a more rational system of long-term care. By focusing on function as being uniquely relevant to the health problems of the elderly and to the goals of long-term services, information about ALE would enable the development of an improved balance in health policies between acute and long-term care. For research, emphasis on function would highlight the need to explore the causes and mechanisms of dysfunction and to develop improved approaches to tertiary prevention. Thus, active life expectancy would contribute to improved care for the elderly and to an enhanced quality of life.

NOTES

1. Katz, S., Branch, L. G., Branson, M. H., Papsidero, J. A., Beck, J. C., and Greer, D. S. Active life expectancy. *New Engl J Med* 309:1218–1224, 1983.

2. Katz, S., and Akpom, C. A. A measure of primary socio-biological functions. *Int J Health Serv* 6:493–508, 1976.

3. Branch, L. G. *Understanding the Health and Social Service Needs of People Over Age 65.* Cambridge, Mass.: Center for Survey Research, Facility of University of Massachusetts and Joint Center for Urban Studies of Massachusetts Institute of Technology and Harvard University, 1977.

4. Shyrock, H. S., and Siegel, J. S. *The Methods and Materials of Demography: The Life Table.* U.S. Bureau of the Census. Washington, D.C.: U.S. Government Printing Office, 1971, pp. 443–446.

5. Ewbank, D., and Wray, J.D. Population and Public Health. In *Maxcy-Rosenau Public Health and Preventive Medicine,* 11th Edition, Last, J. M. ed. New York: Appleton-Century-Crofts, 1980, pp. 1517–1521.

6. Mausner, J. S., and Bahn, A. K. Epidemiology: An Introductory Text. Philadelphia: Saunders, 1974, pp. 198–200 and 307–309.

7. Whittenberger, J. L. The physical and chemical environment. In *Preventive and Community Medicine,* Clark, D. W., and MacMahon, B. eds. Boston: Little, Brown: 1981.

8. Shapiro, S. A tool for health planners. *Am J Public Health* 67:816–817, 1977.

9. Kleinman, J. C. The continued vitality of vital statistics. *Am J Public Health* 72:125–127, 1982.

10. Jenkins, W. A., and Lew, E. A. A new mortality basis for annuities. *Trans Soc Actuaries* 1:369–468, 1949.

11. Bright, M. Demographic background for programming chronic diseases in the United States. In *Chronic Diseases and Public Health,* Lillienfeld, A. M., and Gifford, A. J., eds. Baltimore: Johns Hopkins Press, 1966, pp. 5–23.

12. Patrick, C. H., Palesch, Y. Y., Feinleib, M., and Brody, J. A. Sex differences in declining cohort death rates from heart disease. *Am J Public Health* 72:161–166, 1982.

13. Somers, A. F. Life-style and health. In *Maxcy-Rosenau Public Health and Preventive Medicine,* 11th Edition, Last, J. M., ed. New York: Appleton-Century-Crofts, 1980, pp. 1046–1065.

14. Deevey, E. S. Life tables for natural populations of animals. *Rev Biol* 22:283–314, 1947.

15. Fries, J. F. Aging, natural death, and the compression of morbidity. *N Engl J Med* 303:130–135, 1980.

16. Donabedian, A. Evaluating the quality of medical care. *Milbank Mem Fund Q* 44:166–206, 1966.

17. Collins, S. D. Sickness surveys. In *Administrative Medicine*, Emerson, H., ed. New York: Nelson, 1951.

18. Katz, S., Hedrick, S. C., and Henderson, N. S. The measurement of long-term care needs and impact. *Health Med Care Serv Rev* 2:1–21, 1979.

19. Dorn, H. F. Some problems for research in mortality and morbidity. *Public Health Rep* 71:1–5, 1956.

20. Jackson, E. H. Duration of disabling acute illness among employed males and females: Eastern Health District of Baltimore, 1938–1943. *Milbank Mem Fund Q* 29:294–300, 1951.

21. Dominion Bureau of Statistics and Department of National Health and Welfare. *Canadian Sickness Survey 1950–51, No. 9*. Ottawa: Queen's Printer and Controller of Stationery, 1956, p. 18.

22. Commission on Chronic Illness. *Chronic Illness in the United States, Vol. IV: Chronic Illness in a Large City*. Cambridge, Mass.: Harvard University Press, 1957.

23. National Center for Health Statistics. *Origin, Program, and Operation of the U.S. National Health Survey*. Rockville, Md. PHS Pub. No. 1000, Vital and Health Statistics, Series 1, No. 1, 1963.

24. Katz, S., Akpom, C. A., Papsidero, J. A., and Weiss, S. T. Measuring the health status of populations. In *Health Status Indexes*. Chicago: Hospital Research and Educational Trust, 1973.

25. Kegeles, S. S. Why people seek dental care: A test of conceptual formulation. *J Health Human Behavior* 4:166, 1963.

26. Kalimo, E., Siever, E., Purola, T., and Numan, K. *The Utilization of the Medical Services and Its Relationship to Morbidity, Health Resources, and Social Factors*. Helsinki, Finland: Publications of the National Pensions Institute of Finland, Series A3, Research Institute for Social Security, 1968.

27. Sydenstricker, E., and Wiehl, D. G. A study of the incidence of disabling sickness in a South Carolina cotton mill village in 1918. *Public Health Rep* 39:1723–1738, 1924.

28. Sydenstricker, E. The incidence of illness in a general population group: General results of a morbidity study from December 1, 1921 through March 31, 1924 in Hagerstown, Maryland. *Public Health Rep* 40:279–291, 1925.

29. Perrott, G. St. J., and Collins, S. D. Relation of sickness to income and income change in ten surveyed communities. *Public Health Rep* 50:595–622, 1935.

30. Wiehl, D. G. and Berry, K. Maternal health and supervision in a rural area. *Milbank Mem Fund Q* 17:172, 1939.

31. Downes, J. Causes of illness among males and females. *Milbank Mem Fund Q* 28:407–428, 1950.

32. Downes, J., and Collins, S.D. A study of illness among families in the Eastern Health District of Baltimore. *Milbank Mem Fund Q* 18:5–26, 1940.

33. Collins, S. D., Phillips, F. R., and Oliver, D. S. Disabling illness from specific causes among males and females of various ages. *Public Health Rep* 66:1649–1671, 1951.

34. Downes, J. Method of statistical analysis of chronic disease in a longitudinal study of illness. *Milbank Mem Fund Q* 29:404–422, 1951.

35. Downes, J. The longitudinal study of families as a method of research. *Milbank Mem Fund Q* 30:101–118, 1952.

36. Downes, J., and Keller, M. The risk of disability for persons with chronic disease. *Milbank Mem Fund Q* 30:311–340, 1952.

37. Trussel, R. D., and Elinson, J. Chronic illness in a rural area. *Chronic Illness in the United States, Vol. III: Chronic Illness in a Rural Area.* Cambridge, Mass.: Harvard University Press, 1959.

38. Bright, M. A follow-up study of the Commission on Chronic Illness Morbidity Survey in Baltimore: I. Tracing a large population sample over time. *J Chron Dis* 20:707–716, 1969.

39. Bright, M. A follow-up study of the Commission on Chronic Illness Morbidity Survey in Baltimore: III. Residential mobility and prospective studies. *J Chron Dis* 21:749–759, 1969.

40. Mooney, W. *Methodology in Two California Health Surveys.* Washington, D.C.: U.S. Government Printing Office, Public Health Monograph No. 70, 1962.

41. National Center for Health Statistics. Health Survey Procedure: Concepts. Questionnaire Development, and Definitions in the *Health Interview Survey.* Rockville, Md.: PHS Pub. No. 1000, Vital and Health Statistics, Series 1, No. 2, 1964.

42. National Center for Health Statistics. *Measures of Chronic Illness Among Residents of Nursing and Personal Care Homes.* Rockville, Md.: DHEW Publication No. (HRA) 74-1709, Vital and Health Statistics, Series 12, No. 24.

43. Fanshel, S., and Bush, J. W. A health status index and its application for health services outcomes. *Operation Res* 18:1021–1066, 1970.

44. Lerner, M. The level of physical health of the poverty population: A conceptual reappraisal of structural factors. *Med Care* 6:355–367, 1968.

45. Miller, J. E. An indicator to aid management in assigning program priorities. *Public Health Rep* 85:725–731, 1970.

46. Sullivan, D.F. A single index of mortality and morbidity. *HSMHA Health Rep* 86:347–354, 1971.

47. Jones, E.W., McNitt, B.H., and McKnight, E.M. *Patient Classification for Long-Term Care: User's Manual.* Washington, D.C.: U.S. Government Printing Office, DHEW Publication No. (HRA) 74-3017, 1973.

48. Katz, S., Ford, A. B., Moskowitz, R. W., Jackson, B. A., and Jaffe, M. W. Studies of illness in the aged. The Index of ADL: A standardized measure of biological and psychosocial function. JAMA 185:914–919, 1963.

49. Katz, S., Heiple, K. G., Downs, T. P., Ford, A. B., and Scott, C. P. Long-term course of 147 patients with fracture of the hip. *Surg Gyn Obs* 124:1219–1230, 1967.

50. Katz, S., Ford, A. B., Chinn, A. B., and Newill, V. A. Prognosis after strokes: Part II, Long-term course of 159 patients. *Medicine* 45:236–246, 1966.

51. Katz, S., Vignos, P. J., Jr., Moscowitz, R. W., Thompson, H. M. and Svec, K. H. Comprehensive outpatient care in rheumatoid arthritis: A controlled study. JAMA 206:1249–1254, 1968.

52. Katz, S., Ford, A. B., Downs, T. D., Adams, M., and Rusby, D. I. *Effects of Continued Care: A Study of Chronic Illness in the Home.* Washington, D.C.: U.S. Government Printing Office, DHEW Publication No. (HSM) 73-3010, 1972.

53. Papsidero, J., Katz, S., Kroger, Sr., M. H., and Akpom, C. *Chance for Change.* East Lansing, Mich.: Michigan State University Press, 1979.

54. National Center for Health Statistics. *The National Nursing Home Survey: 1977 Summary for the United States.* Hyattsville, Md.: Public Health Service, DHHS Publication No. (PHS) 79-1794, Vital and Health Statistics, Series 13, No. 43, 1979.

55. Densen, P.M., Jones, E.W., and McNitt, B.J. *An Approach to the Assessment of Long-Term Care: Final Report.* Boston: Harvard Center for Community Health and Medical Care, 1976.

56. Weissert, W., Wan, T., Livieratos, B., and Katz, S. Effects and costs of day-care services for the chronically ill. *Med Care* 18:567–584, 1980.

57. Technical Consultant Panel on the Long-Term Health Care Data Set, U.S. National Committee on Vital and Health Statistics. *Long-Term Health Care: Minimum Data Set. Final Report.* Hyattsville, Md.: National Center for Health Statistics, DHHS Publication No. (PHS) 80-1158, 1979.

58. Fox, P. D., and Clauser, S. B. Trends in nursing home expenditures: Implications for aging policy. *Health Care Financing Rev*, 2(2):65–70.

Health, Disease, and Cardiovascular Aging

Edward G. Lakatta*

As we age, changes in our appearance may be accompanied by changes in the way in which our body organs function. In general, it is felt by many students of gerontology—the study of aging—that progressive functional declines in organ systems occur with advancing age, and on this basis, global (but not readily testable) hypotheses of a "biologic aging process" have been formulated.[1] Upon a casual review of the literature that describes these functional declines in various organ systems, one is struck with the fact that the rate of functional decline varies dramatically among organs and that within a given system, there is a wide scatter among individuals. This implies that some other factor or factors are potent modulators of a "biological clock" that determines how we age. One such factor is the occurrence of specific processes that we have traditionally referred to as disease. At this point in our discussion we might wonder whether we should classify the "aging process" as a disease as well, since, like specific pathologic entities, it too may result in functional decline and eventually in death. However, regardless of what play on language we choose, the two, i.e., disease and aging, must be specifically delineated in order to identify and characterize the latter. This task is not so difficult when a disease process is overt; however,

*Chief, Cardiovascular Section, Gerontology Research Center, National Institute on Aging, Bethesda, Maryland.

the presence of occult disease can cause marked functional impairments and confound the issue.

The interaction of diseases and aging can be considered from multiple perspectives: (a) functional changes due to aging per se interfere with the assessment of the extent or severity of a disease process; (b) aging of an organism modifies its tolerance to pathological states, thus modifying the clinical presentation and prognosis of a disease; and (c) the presence of disease interferes with studies of the pure age affect. The latter consideration is especially pertinent to investigation of the effect of age on the cardiovascular system in humans because the incidence and prevalence of cardiovascular disease, and of coronary atherosclerosis in particular, increase exponentially with age, and as we shall see, these diseases are present in an occult form in a substantial number of elderly persons.

In addition to disease, changes in life style occur concomitantly with advancing age. By this I am referring to habits such as exercise, eating, drinking, smoking, and thinking, which are determined by education, socioeconomic status, and character traits. These life style variables are particularly important because they can be modified, and if they can alter an "aging process," or prevent a disease process, we would certainly like to know about it. Indeed, though our understanding is very far from complete, over the past two decades we have become aware of the impact of smoking, nutritional, behavioral, and possibly physical activity "habits" on the clinical manifestations of coronary artery disease. The impact of life style on the aging process, on the other hand, is at present less well defined, and it is likely that many changes in cardiovascular function that have previously been attributed to an aging process were in part due to the sedentary life style that accompanies aging.

Given the fact that, with advancing age, the prevalence of disease increases sharply and major changes in life style occur, and considering that aging, disease, and life style are intertwined, elucidation of the presence and nature of an aging process is a formidable task; extrapolation of the notion of an aging process in the cardiovascular system to a theory of aging at the present time borders on absurdity.

A very different approach toward eventually defining an aging process begins by attempting to control for disease and life style, then defines which functional alterations, if any, occur with advancing age in various organ systems, and then proceeds to study the underlying mechanism for each of the functional deficits. Should these mechanisms be similar among organ systems, a global aging "process" might legitimately be defined. In this paper it is my aim to examine the age-related changes within the cardiovascular system that such an approach has defined.

VASCULAR DISEASE AND AGING

Atherosclerosis is usually perceived as a problem of advanced age. This is something of a misconception. A more precise statement regarding these vascular changes that occur with age is that the disease process begins at a young age but its *severity* increases progressively over the entire adult age span, and when a critical stage is reached, the abnormality becomes noticeable to an individual or to his or her physician.

The term "hardening of the arteries" is rather broad and includes changes in the vascular surface in contact with blood (the intima), in the middle part or muscular coat of the vessel (the media), and in the outer fibrous layer of the large or central, cerebral, peripheral, and coronary arteries, i.e., the blood vessels that supply the heart itself. Just how often these arterial disease processes are present (i.e., their prevalence), and how often they are likely to be severe enough to be diagnosed as a medical problem can be ascertained by considering the combined results of studies implemented both during life and at necropsy.

Over a period of 5 years (1960–1965), the International Atherosclerosis Project collected vascular specimens from approximately 24,000 men and women comprising 19 geographical–race groups.[2] The specimens were graded for different manifestations of intimal pathology. These included fibrous plaques (areas of scarring due to the atherosclerotic process), deposition of calcium, and the extent of narrowing (stenosis) of the vessel caused by these abnormalities. The prevalence of fibrous plaques, calcific lesions, and stenosis in coronary arteries in a sample from a New Orleans Caucasian population is presented in Figure 1. The first point of interest in the figure is that early manifestations of this disease, i.e., fibrous plaques, are present in 30 percent of hearts from individuals between the ages of 15 and 24 years, and that by ages 35 to 44, more than 85 percent of hearts demonstrate this abnormality. Also apparent is the increase in the presence

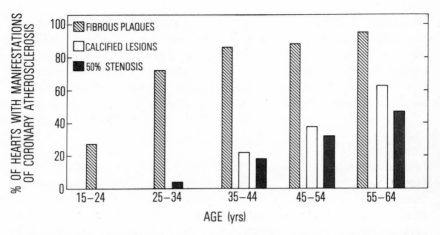

FIGURE 1 Manifestations of atherosclerosis in coronary arteries from hearts of individuals of a New Orleans Caucasian population. The data for fibrosis and calcific lesions were derived from those individuals who died from accidents, infections, and miscellaneous causes other than heart disease. Data for stenotic lesions were derived from individuals of this population who died from any cause. Redrawn from Tejada et al.[2]

of calcification with age; by age 55 to 64, over 60 percent of hearts exhibit vascular calcification.

Given this marked age-related increase in fibrous and calcific vascular lesions, a substantial case might be made for defining these changes as "aging," rather than denoting them as a disease called atherosclerosis. The distinction, however, would be largely semantic. Perhaps the most potent argument against attributing atherosclerosis to an aging process is the fact that 50 percent of all deaths in western countries are due to myocardial infarction (heart attacks) and cerebral infarctions (strokes). In most instances the death of an individual is caused by a lack of blood supply to the heart and brain, while these organs themselves (as we shall see below for the heart) are still capable of maintaining a high level of function. That the vessels supplying an organ should "age" out of phase with the organ they supply seems teleologically unsound. Rather, in the context of the efficiency of our existence, it makes more sense to consider the process demonstrated by the data in Figure 1 as a disease rather than as aging per se.

Coronary artery atherosclerosis can modify myocardial function, which we will attempt to assess in order to identify the presence of age-related changes, by reducing myocardial blood flow. Thus, the most important vascular abnormality to consider in this regard is not the presence of fibrous or calcific lesions, but rather vessel narrowing or stenosis. Figure 1 illustrates that the prevalence of vessel narrowing also increases with age, so that by ages 55 to 64, half of all hearts studied had 50 percent or more occlusion in at least one of the three major coronary arteries. In a similar autopsy study in Rochester, Minnesota, performed in the mid-1950s, it was found that 60 to 70 percent of subjects in this age range or older who died from all causes had significant (50 to 60 percent) narrowing of at least one major artery.[3,4]

Although a high percentage of elderly individuals have stenosis at autopsy, a much lower percentage have clinical symptoms; in other words, the disease is in an occult stage during life in a large number of individuals. It is imperative to detect the occult form of this disease in order to determine whether interventions such as a change in life style variables will have an impact on its progression, or to develop pharmacological therapeutics in an attempt to retard its progression. It is particularly important to detect its presence when investigating the impact of an aging process in the myocardium, since heart function, particularly during stress, is highly dependent on coronary blood flow.

Recent technological advances have been made in radionuclide imaging of the myocardium, i.e., in obtaining a picture of the heart after it has taken up a radioactive substance. This technique, coupled with electrocardiographic monitoring during an exercise stress on the cardiovascular system, has helped identify many individuals with "occult" coronary disease. The principle on which these tests are based is relatively simple. With exercise, the heart, performing more work, requires additional oxygen and therefore an increased supply of blood. Normally, the coronary arterial system reduces its resistance during exercise and permits greater blood flow. A stenotic lesion, e.g., due to atherosclerosis, as discussed above, represents a fixed narrowing and thus interferes with augmentation of blood supply during exercise, resulting in a relative deficiency of oxygen delivery to the area of the heart supplied by that vessel. This relative lack of blood flow, or ischemia, often manifests itself as an abnormality in the electrocardiogram (ECG). A more direct determination of relative

ischemia than can be made from the ECG is provided by the
radioactive tracer method. One such tracer is thallous ion, which,
when injected into the vascular system, will be evenly distributed
throughout the heart; its radiation can then be measured by a
gamma camera. In a person who has coronary artery stenosis
that is not so severe as to limit blood supply at rest, when the
heart is working minimally, the heart image will be normal.
During exercise, when the demand for blood flow in the area
supplied by the stenotic vessel exceeds the supply, that area will
appear as a "cold spot" relative to other areas on the image of
the heart in which blood supply has increased normally. The
potential effectiveness of these two relatively noninvasive techniques, electrocardiography and thallium scanning, during exercise in screening for occult coronary disease is demonstrated
in Figure 2. The lower shaded area indicates the prevalence of
coronary disease as estimated by the usual epidemiologic techniques, i.e., history of myocardial infarction or angina pectoris,

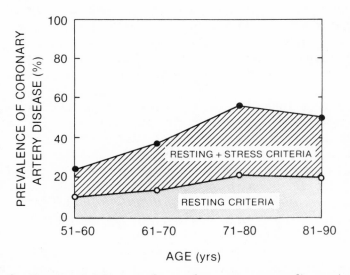

AGE (yrs)

FIGURE 2   Estimate of the prevalence of coronary artery disease in men
aged 51 to 90. Subjects were participants in the Baltimore Longitudinal
Study of Aging. Resting criteria are history of angina pectoris or myocardial
infarction, or an abnormal ECG at rest; stress criteria are the presence of
an abnormal ECG (J point depression of at least 1 mm and flat S-T segment
for at least .04 s) or a thallium scan perfusion defect during exercise, or
both. Redrawn from Gerstenblith et al.[5]

and/or an abnormal resting ECG. The addition of stress criteria, i.e., ECG or thallium scan abnormalities during exercise, doubles the estimate of the prevalence of coronary disease in these men of middle and advanced age (hatched area); this estimate approaches the known prevalence based on autopsy studies (Figure 1). As we shall see, recent studies of the effect of age on cardiovascular physiology in subjects screened for coronary disease by this method yield some radically different results from previous studies in populations in which the presence of hidden coronary disease was not sought or detected.

While we have focused on changes in the intima and subintima of the coronary arteries, changes also occur in the medial layers of vessels with advancing age. These include changes in the amount or character of elastin (elastic-like fibers) and collagen (connective tissue), as well as an accumulation of calcium. The precise relationship of these changes to those occurring in the intima has not yet been established. Over the past several decades attention has focused on the lipid diet theory as a major causal factor in the intimal atherosclerotic process. However, since the intimal processes are paralleled by those in the media,[6] it has been suggested by some scientists that the two may be a common manifestation of vascular aging. It is hoped that research over the next several decades will investigate this notion in some detail, since it may be critical to understanding treating the atherosclerotic process.

The alterations that occur in the vessel media with aging are the apparent cause of the increased stiffness of blood vessels noted to accompany advancing age. Although these changes, unlike the intimal changes described above, do not usually produce severe vascular narrowing or clinical disease, they do affect cardiac function in that they may alter the resistance to blood flowing from the heart to the periphery. Consider that the heart, in pumping blood, "forces" it through the vessels. With each heart beat the large vessels expand somewhat to accommodate the blood. Stiffer vessels are less accommodating, and when an equivalent volume of blood is pumped into them, the resulting pressure will be higher than in normal arteries. The heart will have to do more work to pump out its blood into a higher pressure system (see below).

In addition to these anatomical changes in vascular media, alterations in function of the smooth muscle also occur with advancing age and may alter cardiovascular performance. During exercise, catecholamine secretion regulates vascular smooth muscle tone and results in differential blood flow to various organs. A diminished vascular responsiveness to catecholamines (adrenalin-like substances) accompanies advancing age and may be implicated in the age-related changes in cardiovascular function during exercise.

LIFE STYLE VARIABLES

While certain types of habits, for example, smoking, diet, and behavior, have been demonstrated to be associated statistically with the clinical manifestations of coronary heart disease and stroke, as noted above, our current understanding of the precise interaction of life style variables, aging, and disease is rather superficial. One reason for this is the difficulty in quantifying these life style variables and measuring them repeatedly. Thus, in 1984, such questions as Will optimal nutrition retard aging? or Will chronic exercise retard aging or prevent or ameliorate coronary disease? cannot be answered with any degree of certainty. However, it is known for certain that the average daily level of physical activity has a marked impact on cardiovascular function. The raison d'être of the cardiovascular system is to act as a "slave" to the other organs of the body, i.e., to deliver nutrients and other substances in the blood to body organs, to circulate blood cells, and to maintain a constant temperature for cellular function. In the absence of cardiovascular disease these needs are *efficiently* met, nothing more, nothing less. With exercise, cardiac, respiratory, and tissue metabolic systems all increase their level of function from that in the resting state. We may refer to this as "short-range" cardiovascular control. "Long-range control" also exists—that is, these systems chronically adapt their level of function to efficiently provide average daily requirements. In other words, these systems can become in or out of "shape" or "condition" as required. This is illustrated in Figure 3, which depicts the effects of bed rest and subsequent conditioning on maximum cardiac output in five different individuals. Note that bed rest can cause up to a 40 percent reduction in maximum output and that this can be reversed by regular physical activity. Because the magnitude of the conditioning effect can be so great, in studies which attempt to investigate to what extent a disease or an "aging process" alters cardiovascular func-

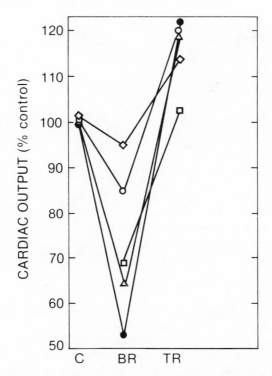

FIGURE 3 Effect of a 21-day bed rest period followed by a 60-day period of moderate physical training on maximum cardiac output in five healthy young volunteer subjects. C, control prior to bed rest (BR); TR, physical training. Redrawn from Saltin et al.[7]

tion (particularly reserve function), the physical activity status must be either controlled for or considered when interpreting the results. This is of particular importance in examining the effect of age, since it has been well established that the average daily physical activity level declines progressively with age in unselected populations;[8] the same was true in a subset of participants in the Baltimore Longitudinal Study of Aging (BLSA) (Figure 4), who were free of coronary disease as judged from the resting-plus-stress criteria in Figure 2. The magnitude of this age effect is likely to be greater in chronically institutionalized subjects than in independent community dwellers.[10] This might seriously hamper the interpretation of studies seeking to define an age effect in institutionalized populations.

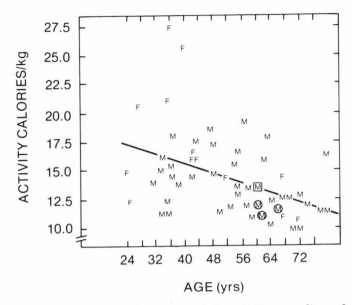

AGE (yrs)

FIGURE 4   Effect of age on the average daily caloric expenditure for physical activity in male (M) and female (F) participants in the Baltimore Longitudinal Study of Aging who were judged free from coronary disease on the basis of resting and stress criteria given in Figure 2. Circles indicate overlap of two males; the square is an overlap of one male and female. Activity calories/kg = 20.09 − 0.11 (age), $r = .46, p < .001$. Redrawn from Rodeheffer et al.[9]

"BIOLOGICAL AGING" OF CARDIOVASCULAR FUNCTION

Given the difficulty of controlling for multiple life style variables and excluding the presence of occult coronary vascular disease, it is fair to say that a perfect study to determine the nature of an aging process within the cardiovascular system (or possibly in any system) remains to be implemented. Rather, most studies have described differences in younger versus older men in selected populations and these differences could be related to aging, to life style, or to disease, or to interactions among these factors.

The cardiovascular system functions over a wide range of performance, often quantitated as cardiac output. Basal or resting cardiac output is approximately one-third to one-sixth the maximum, and a basal output of 40 percent (caused, for example, by a disease) for extended periods of time is usually not compatible with life. By convention, cardiac output is expressed in L/min (or L/min/m², i.e., cardiac index) and is determined by the product of the volume of blood ejected in each beat (stroke volume) and the number of beats per minute (heart rate). Both stroke volume and heart rate are controlled by neuronal and hormonal influences; in addition, stroke volume depends on the level of excitation–contraction coupling (contractile state), the venous return to the heart between beats (preload), and the impedance to ventricular ejection (afterload). The contractile state, preload, and afterload are interdependent, and each of these is influenced by neurohormonal modulation. Another factor, coronary flow, modulates the contractile state and is influenced not only by the integrity of the coronary vasculature, as discussed above, and by neurohormonal modulation, but also by the pre- and afterload and the duration of the diastolic filling period. Thus, cardiac output is determined by a number of interdependent factors and a weakness in any one, for example, as a result of a disease or aging process, leads to compensatory alterations in others which may return overall function—cardiac output—toward normal. Thus, while the description of a biologic aging process is made difficult because of the interaction of aging, disease, and life style, the precise definition of an abnormal hemodynamic variable is also a formidable task. Each of the following factors—heart rate, intrinsic cell performance, load prior to shortening, load during shortening, and coronary flow—is ultimately regulated by cellular Ca^{2+} metabolism and other molecular mechanisms. When a true age-related change in a particular factor is defined, the next step toward defining an aging process is to elucidate the molecular mechanism involved. This mandates the use of animal aging models.

DOES AN AGING PROCESS MODIFY CARDIAC OUTPUT AT REST?

Many gerontologists believe that basal cardiac output declines progressively over the adult age range (Figure 5A), and have suggested that this is a manifestation of an aging process within the cardiovascular system. However, a recent study contrasts sharply with this view. In that study (Figure 5B), cardiac output at rest did not decline with age over a comparable age range to that studied in panel A. While the heart rate in the populations

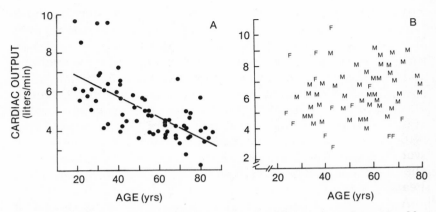

FIGURE 5   A. The relation between age and cardiac output, determined by the Direct Fick method in 67 "basal" males without apparent circulatory disorders. The line indicates a significant linear regression for the points. From Brandfonbrener et al.[11] B. The effect of age on cardiac output at rest determined by radionuclide angiography in subjects from the Baltimore Longitudinal Study of Aging. See text for details. M, males; F, females. From Rodeheffer et al.[9] Figures 5A and 5B reprinted by permission of the American Heart Association, Inc.

shown in both A and B tended to be lower with advancing age, the major factor associated with the decreased cardiac output in population A was an age-related decrease in stroke volume that did not occur in population B. This result poses a formidable challenge to the notion of the occurrence of an aging process that mandates an irreversible progressive decline in cardiac output with age, over this age range at least. When the literature on aging is considered as a whole, studies that investigated an effect of age on cardiac performance fail to demonstrate a unique age effect on resting cardiac output[12,13]; this suggests that an effect of age on cardiac output at rest likely does not exist, but rather that age-related trends observed in basal cardiac output depend on the particular population studied.

The results of the two studies in Figure 5 represent the extreme estimates of the effect of age on cardiac output at rest.[13] The subject population in Figure 5A was comprised of patients from both the acute and chronic wards of a community hospital, none of whom had histories or physical signs compatible with cardiovascular disease. However, many were convalescing from either surgical procedures, respiratory infections, or orthopedic conditions. The subject population in Figure 5B was comprised of participants of the BLSA.[9] More specifically, this particular subset was comprised of consecutive volunteers in whom signs and symptoms of cardiovascular disease were absent; resting and stress ECG were normal; for those over the age of 40, stress thallium images were also normal. It is important to note, however, that even in this population, estimates of physical activity as judged from the average daily caloric expenditure for activity[8] declined with age (Figure 4). Thus, the elderly participants in this study were not "conditioned" with regard to physical activity prior to the study as an athlete might be, but rather represented average healthy community dwellers.

Although the study in panel A of Figure 5 was more heavily weighted on both age extremes than that in panel B, the marked differences between the two over the ages of 30 to 80 cannot be attributed to a different age range or to different methodologies for measuring cardiac output. While the difference between panels A and B could be due to some unspecified cohort effect, a more attractive hypothesis is that it resulted, at least in part, from differences in the extent of occult coronary disease and in the physical conditioning status of institutionalized versus community dwellers. It must be noted that both studies A and B were cross-sectional in design, i.e., different individuals of different ages were compared. It might be argued that in either study, different results might have prevailed had the study design been longitudinal, i.e., if each subject had been followed across the entire age span and each serial measurement compared to earlier ones in that individual. To date, no such studies of cardiac output or function have been implemented. The technique used to study population B, however, lends itself to this type of design in that it is as accurate as the technique used in A but is relatively noninvasive.

Additional caution in interpreting the results in Figure 5B as being indicative of the absence of an "age effect" is warranted by the fact that this study examined adult age only up to 80 years. It would be truly unwise to linearly extrapolate the results of any study of aging past the last measured data point because (a) a true aging process might not become manifest until a later age than that studied, or (b) even when an age effect is observed over the age range studied, the slope of that function may change markedly with further aging.

While a unique effect of age on basal cardiac output has not been obtained in several investigations of that question, a result that has been virtually universally obtained (when sufficient numbers across a broad enough age range have been studied) is that systolic blood pressure increases progressively with age. This has been true both in cross-sectional and longitudinal analyses as well.[14] The basal systolic blood pressure in the subjects in Figure 5B is depicted in Figure 6A. Note that this age-related change in blood pressure occurs *within* the limit that medical scientists have arbitrarily defined as the "normal" range of blood pressure. High blood pressure or "hypertension" in the elderly, i.e., blood pressure outside this designated normal clinical range, is another matter, and may be attributed to other factors in addition to the stiffening of the large arteries with age discussed above.

This increase in systolic blood pressure imposes an increased work load on the heart during each beat (Figure 6B). The extent of the shortening of myocardial fibers, which determines the volume of blood ejected during a heart beat, varies inversely with the stress or load the myofilaments bear. When marked increases in work load are imposed on the myocardium, as in the disease states of severe hypertension or valvular heart disease, the heart wall thickens markedly and normalizes the load or myocardial wall stress, which is determined by force per unit area of the myocardial wall. This wall thickening facilitates the ejection of blood during each beat in these disease states. A mild increase in myocardial wall thickness with advancing age would, in a similar fashion, be an adaptive mechanism to normalize the moderate increase in myocardial wall stress imposed by the higher systolic pressure. Conversely, a failure to increase myocardial wall thickness (hypertrophy) in response to this enhanced work load might indeed be referred to as a manifestation of an aging process. Whether the myocardium hypertrophies with advancing age has until recently been a rather controversial subject, and the concept that the heart undergoes atrophy rather than hypertrophy in advanced age has been advocated.[15] This notion is by no means universally held, however. In fact, the data accumulated in many studies indicate that, in humans, the heart hypertrophies with advancing age.[16] However, hearts from individuals with cardiovascular disease, who, as noted, increase in number sharply with age, were included with hearts from normal individuals in reaching this conclusion.

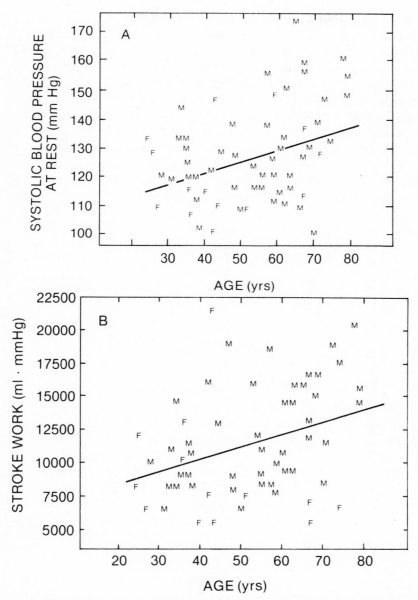

FIGURE 6 Effect of age on (A) basal systolic blood pressure and (B) stroke work, defined as the product of systolic pressure and stroke volume, in the Baltimore Longitudinal Study of Aging participants depicted in Figures 4 and 5B. Systolic blood pressure (mm Hg) = 105.26 + 0.41 (age), r = .37, $p < .003$. Stroke work (ml · mm Hg) = 6451 + 98 (age), r = .36, $p < .004$. M, males; F, females. Reconstructed from Rodeheffer et al.[9]

The presence of cardiac hypertrophy has been sought nonin-
vasively in living healthy men by echocardiography; Figure 7
illustrates that an age-related increase in left ventricle wall
thickness between the ages of 25 to 80 years has been identified.
(The population examined in Figure 7 was a subset of the BLSA,
screened in essentially the same manner as the subjects in Figure
5B.) In this same study, advancing age was associated with a
reduced rate of ventricular filling, which in part contributed to
the wall thickening observed with age. Similar significant but
less marked age-related changes also occur in women.[18] It is not
inconceivable that cardiac atrophy with aging might be observed
in chronically institutionalized populations, in whom multiple

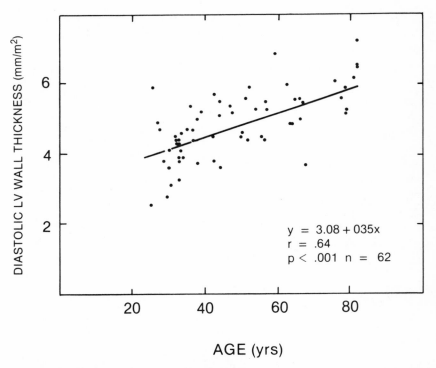

AGE (yrs)

FIGURE 7   Linear regression plot depicting the relationship between age
and diastolic left ventricular (LV) wall thickness/m^2 in male participants
in the Baltimore Longitudinal Study of Aging. Increased age is associated
with increased diastolic wall thickness. From Gerstenblith et al.[17] Reprinted
by permission of the American Heart Association, Inc.

diseases are present. However, this cannot be attributed to aging per se.

CARDIOVASCULAR RESPONSE TO STRESS

That basal cardiac output is not altered by age in healthy active subjects by no means indicates that cardiovascular performance during stress is unaffected by advancing age. In fact, among the earliest manifestations of an aging process would be a loss of functional reserve. In order to detect this, a given organ system must be stressed to the maximum extent. Classical studies in exercise physiology have indicated that maximum exercise tolerance diminishes with age in apparently healthy persons.[13] Specifically, age-related decline has been identified in maximum aerobic capacity, heart rate, stroke volume, cardiac output, and arteriovenous oxygen differences. A result that typifies such studies is given in Figure 8A.

One important aspect of comparisons of maximum cardiac function in different aged subjects is that these comparisons are sometimes made not at standard exercise levels across all ages, but at the voluntary maximal exercise level of each subject, which is usually substantially reduced with age. In Figure 8A, for example, since no plateau in the curves is evident, it cannot be ascertained whether maximum cardiac performance was achieved in the elderly, or whether the limitation in exercise tolerance with advanced age might be due to other factors. In this regard, consideration of the impact of occult coronary diseases is even more important in studies during exercise than in studies of the cardiovascular system at rest. In fact, an age-dependent increase in ECG abnormalities during exercise, which in some instances may be indicative of coronary disease, has been observed in previous studies.[20,21] Furthermore, the status of physical conditioning is also a major determinant of the exercise response.[22] Figure 8B depicts the exercise response of the BLSA subjects studied at rest in Figure 5B. Comparison of Figures 8A and 8B demonstrates, as in the case of studies at rest, that extremely different results can be obtained in different populations. While in these BLSA subjects the maximum work load achieved declined with age, this decline was significantly less marked than in Figure 8A (compare the cardiac outputs achieved in both panels); thus, the physical endurance of the elderly in this population was ap-

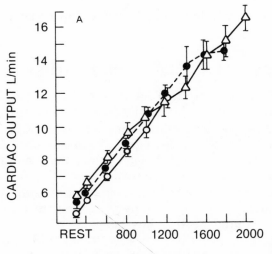

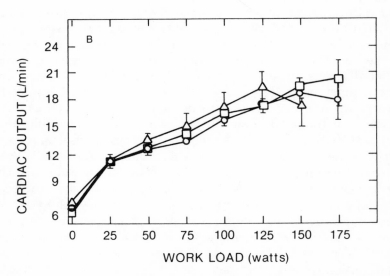

FIGURE 8 A. Cardiac output in 54 apparently healthy subjects (35 males and 19 females) aged 18–34 (△), 35–49 (●), and 50–69 years of age (○). Increasing levels of oxygen consumption represent increasing work loads during upright bicycle exercise. With increasing work load, subjects in each group dropped out and the last recorded work load is that in which at least six subjects in each age group participated. STPD: standard temperature, pressure, dry. Redrawn from Julius et al.[19] B. Cardiac output measured during graded upright bicycle exercise in subjects from the Baltimore Lon-

parently greater than in the subjects in Figure 8A and in other previous studies of the effect of age on the exercise response.[13]

While maximum cardiac output in the subjects in Figure 8B did not decline with age, the ability of the heart to function as a pump was affected by age in that the extent to which the left ventricle emptied during each beat was reduced: end-systolic volume increased, and the ejection fraction, or the proportion of end-diastolic volume that is ejected in each stroke, diminished with advancing age. Studies utilizing a similar technique to measure ejection fraction have indicated that, during exercise, the ejection fraction decreases from the resting level in subjects with coronary artery disease.[23] More recently, it has been suggested that a reduction in ejection fraction with exercise could also be attributed to aging per se (Figure 9A). In the BLSA population (Figure 8B), screened for study as noted above, even though the ejection fraction did not increase to the same extent in the elderly as it did in younger subjects, a *reduction* in ejection fraction during exercise from that at the basal level was rarely observed (Figure 9B). This is yet another example of the different results obtained in populations screened for study by different criteria.

This pattern of maintained maximum cardiac output (Figure 8B) in the presence of a diminution in heart rate (see below) and a reduction in some aspects of pump function (higher end-systolic volume, decreased ejection fraction) is indicative of compensatory changes in other factors that regulate cardiac output in elderly subjects. Stated in other words, in healthy elderly subjects an adaptation occurs to prevent a substantial decrease in maximum cardiac output in the presence of a diminished heart rate and diminished pump function. Since cardiac output results from the interplay of several factors, a given increment in cardiac output over the basal level can be achieved with some degree of variability in the extent to which each of these factors changes. Consider the two examples in Figure 10. With increasing work load during exercise, the subject in panel A exhibits a progressive

---

gitudinal Study of Aging. The 61 subjects studied at rest (Figure 5B) have been divided into three age groups for comparison with study in Figure 8A. Group 1 (□) = 25–44 years of age (n = 24); Group II (○) = 45–64 years (n = 21); and Group III (△) = 65–80 years (n = 16). Like the study in panel A, the number of participants in each group decreased with increasing work load.

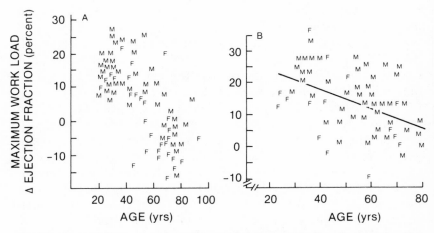

FIGURE 9   A. Effect of age on change in left ventricular ejection fraction from resting level to that at maximum voluntary exercise in apparently healthy subjects. From Port et al.[24] B. Effect of age on change in left ventricular ejection fraction from resting level to that at maximum voluntary exercise in subjects from the Baltimore Longitudinal Study of Aging. M, males; F, females. Rodeheffer et al.[9]

increment in heart rate to approximately 190 beats/min, and while slight dilatation of the heart occurs at low work loads, with increasing loads the heart size is reduced—the end-diastolic or filling volume decreases and the end-systolic volume does so as well. Note also that stroke volume decreases with the fall in end-diastolic volume. The net result is a cardiac output of about 19 L/min. The subject in panel B achieves a similar cardiac output during exercise. Note, however, that in doing so, the heart rate increased to only 130 beats/min. Note also that this subject's heart remained enlarged during exercise, i.e., at all work loads end-diastolic volume remained increased and stroke volume also remained increased over resting levels. Since cardiac output is the product of stroke volume and heart rate, the enhanced stroke volume compensated for a diminished heart rate and cardiac output was maintained at the level of subject A.

The effect of age on the hemodynamic pattern used to augment cardiac output during exercise can be ascertained by examining Figure 11. Note that with advancing age, while the heart rate increase with each progressive increment in work load is less (panel A), the end-diastolic volume (panel B) and stroke volume

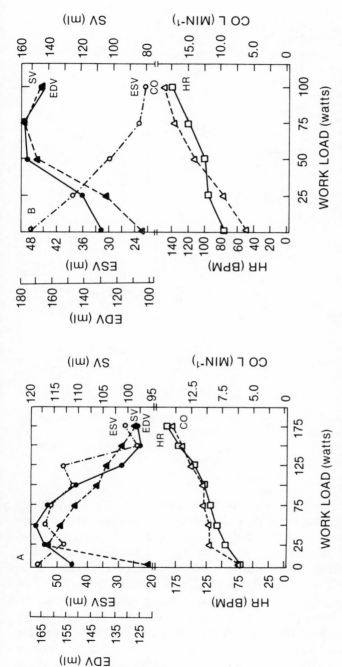

FIGURE 10 Hemodynamic response to graded upright bicycle exercise in two subjects. Note that the same high cardiac output (CO) is obtained by different patterns in panels A and B. In A, heart rate (HR) increased substantially more than in B, while in B, end-diastolic (EDV) and stroke volume (ESV, SV) increased more than in A. BPM, beats/min.

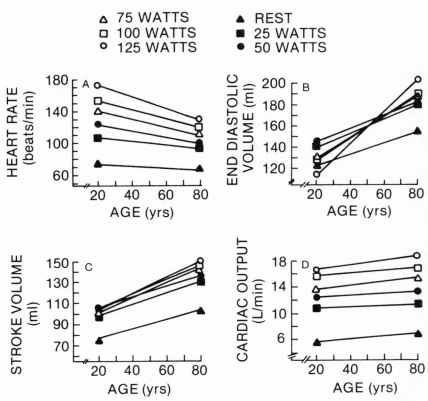

FIGURE 11   The effect of age on heart rate (A), end-diastolic volume (B), stroke volume (C), cardiac output (D), during graded exercise. The number of subjects at each work load is essentially that at rest (see Figure 10; work loads: at rest through work load at 100 watts).

(panel C) increase to greater extents. The net result is that cardiac output does not decline with age (panel D) even in the presence of a diminished heart rate. The essence of the age-related alterations in the hemodynamic pattern of augmented cardiac output is the shift in the slopes of the age regression lines with increasing work load in Figure 11. To illustrate this even more clearly, the slope of the age regression for each parameter in Figure 11 has been plotted as a function of work load in Figure 12. Note that while the slope for heart rate declines, those for end-diastolic volume and stroke volume increase; that for cardiac output remains flat. Note also that the slope for end-systolic volume increases so that the ejection fraction does not increase, and at 100 watts, it actually decreases. Note also that the slope of the age regression for systolic blood pressure does not increase with increasing exercise in this population; this differs from results found in other populations, such as that in Figure 8A.[19]

The age-related alterations in the hemodynamic profile during exercise (Figures 11 and 12) are remarkably similar to those observed when the receptors of beta-adrenergic catecholamines are blocked during exercise. Recall that each of the determinants of cardiac output is subject to autonomic modulation. During exercise, the adrenergic component becomes dominant while the cholinergic influence wanes. The secretion of catecholamines increases during exercise and in part causes an increase in the heart rate; the large arteries[25] as well as arterioles dilate, and

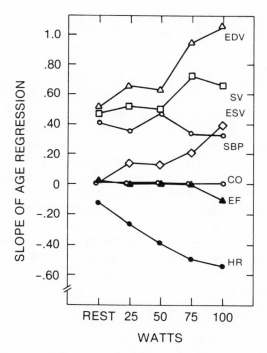

FIGURE 12 Effect of incremental upright bicycle exercise on the slope of the age regression of end-diastolic volume (EDV), stroke volume (SV), end-systolic volume (ESV), heart rate (HR), ejection fraction (EF), cardiac output (CO), and systolic blood pressure (SBP) in the same participants from the Baltimore Longitudinal Study of Aging as in Figures 8B, 9B, and 11.

an increase in the level of excitation–contraction coupling or contractility occurs, resulting in an augmentation of ejection fraction and a reduction in end systolic volume. The extent to which catecholamine secretion occurs during exercise can be ascertained from measurements of serum catecholamine levels, a typical example of which is depicted in Figure 13A. A relative failure of the elaboration of catecholamines during exercise could be a plausible explanation for the observed pattern of altered hemodynamics during exercise with aging. However, this is not the case. In fact, serum levels of catecholamines are increased with age during exercise (Figure 13B). This suggests that the target organ responses to a given level of catecholamines are decreased, or, stated in other words, that the atrial pacemaker, myocardial, and vascular responses at or distal to the beta-receptor appear to decline with advancing age.

There is ample experimental evidence both in human beings and in animal models to support this hypothesis.[27] An age difference in cardiac output noted in a given population prior to pharmacologic beta-blockade was lessened in the presence of beta-blockade.[28] Direct intravenous bolus infusion of isoproterenol, a synthetic beta-adrenergic agonist, causes less of an increment in heart rate in elderly versus younger adult men (Figure 14). In addition, the *maximum* heart rate elicited by such an infusion is substantially reduced in senescent versus younger adult beagle dogs, while electrical pacing results in equal increments in heart rate in young and old dogs alike.[30] Also, in the beagle dog aging model during exercise, the senescent but not the young dogs exhibited an increment in aortic vascular impedance; in the presence of beta-adrenergic blockade by propranolol both young and old dogs exhibited increased aortic vascular impedance, suggesting that this results from a failure of beta-mediated relaxation of aortic smooth muscle.[25] Indeed, direct application of isoproterenol elicits marked relaxation in aortic contracted muscle from young rats and rabbits and only a minor extent of relaxation in muscle from older animals, while nonadrenergic relaxants such as nitroglycerin are equally effective in all age groups studied.[31]

At the cellular level, e.g., the myocardial cell, the beta-adrenergic effect is mediated via a cascade of biochemical events (Figure 15) which effect a change in cell Ca^{2+} metabolism and result

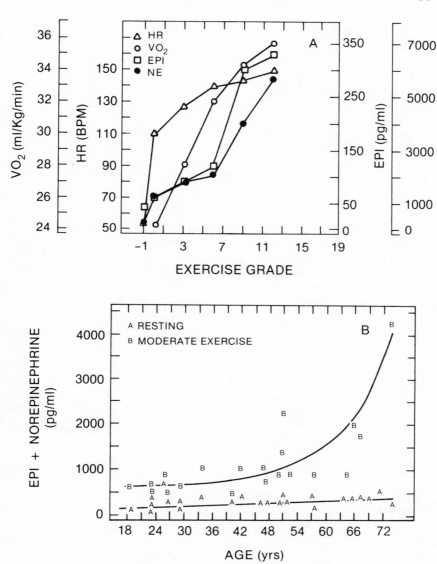

FIGURE 13   A. Rise in heart rate (HR), oxygen consumption (VO$_2$), plasma epinephrine (EPI), and norepinephrine (NE) as a function of graded treadmill exercise. B. Effect of age on plasma catecholamine levels at rest (A) and during moderate exercise levels (B) in Baltimore Longitudinal Study of Aging participants screened for study with prior stress ECG monitoring. From Tzankoff et al.[26]

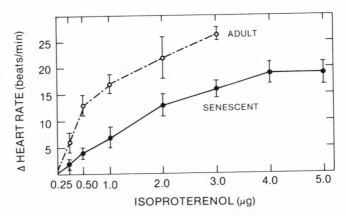

FIGURE 14   Effect of age on the increase in heart rate in response to vary-
ing concentrations of isoproterenol in Baltimore Longitudinal Study of Ag-
ing participants screened as in Figure 13B. Points indicate mean ± SEM.
At all concentrations above 0.5 μg, the effect of age is significant at $p < .005$.
Adult age: 18–34 years, n = 16; senescent age: = 62–80 years, n = 20.
Redrawn from Yin et al.[29]

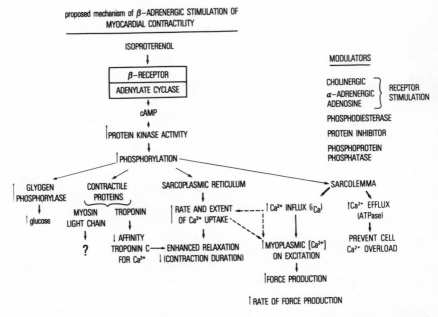

FIGURE 15   Relationship of beta-adrenergically mediated changes in cellular biochemical reactions to enhancement of contractility in cardiac muscle. Reprinted, with permission, from Filburn and Lakatta.[32]

in enhanced contractile performance. The effect of age on some of the steps in Figure 15 has been investigated in an attempt to elucidate the mechanism for the age-related decline in the beta-adrenergically induced increase in force or rate of force production observed in the rat myocardium (Figure 16A). The findings that the beta-receptor characteristics are unaltered and that the increment in 3',5'-cyclic adenosine monophosphate (cAMP) concentration and activation of protein kinase in response to isoproterenol are also not age-related[33] suggest that the mechanism for the age effect in Figure 16A is distal to the protein kinase step in Figure 15. This is supported by the additional observation that dibutyryl cAMP, which does not require an interaction with the receptor or the cell surface or a stimulation of adenylate cyclase, also results in a diminished contractile response in senescent myocardium (Figure 16B). Furthermore, the direct response of the senescent heart to an increase in perfusate $[Ca^{2+}]$,

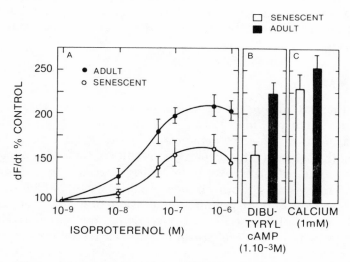

FIGURE 16   A. Effect of age on response of the maximum rate of force development, dF/dt, to isoproterenol in arterially perfused interventricular septa from adult (7–9 mo) and senescent (25 mo) rats. An age difference in dose-response curves of dF/dt is significant at $p < .005$ level (regression analysis of variance, n = 6 in each age group at each isoproterenol concentration). Prior to isoproterenol, dF/dt was not age-related. B. The contractile response to dibutyryl cAMP is diminished in senescent versus adult septa (C). The response to an increment in perfusate $[Ca^{2+}]$ is preserved in the senescent septa. From Guarnieri et al.[33]

which is the final common mediator of enhanced contractility (Figure 15), is not altered by age (Figure 16C and ref. 34). While the precise mechanism for the diminished beta-adrenergic response remains to be demonstrated, these results suggest that age differences in the extent of phosphorylation of various cellular organelles (Figure 15), or in the change in Ca^{2+} metabolism resulting from a given extent of phosphorylation, likely differ with age. A more detailed investigation of these processes in the myocardium,[32] as well as dissection of a similar cascade which mediates the beta-adrenergic response in vascular muscle and the sino-atrial node, are required for the determination of the precise molecular mechanism(s) of the age effect in each of these tissues. If the mechanism is the same in each of them, a diminution in beta-adrenergic response would truly constitute an aging process in the cardiovascular system. Similar studies of tissues from other organs could be compared with those in the cardiovascular system to determine if a diminution in the beta-adrenergic response is a *universal* effect of aging. Additional studies might determine whether this can be reversed by physical "conditioning."

SUMMARY

Studies examining the effect of advanced age on cardiovascular function have provided varied results, ranging from a marked reduction to no change, depending on the criteria used for selecting the subjects. This disparity of results in itself argues against the existence of an irreversible "aging process" that is unique among individuals. Both changes in life style that occur with advancing age and the profound increase in prevalence of stenotic coronary vascular disease with advancing age, particularly the occult form of the disease, present obstacles to studies attempting to demonstrate the presence and nature of an aging process in the cardiovascular system. Certainly if one considers atherosclerosis a manifestation of aging rather than a disease, the task becomes somewhat easier. However, since intrinsic myocardial function is fairly well preserved with age, the changes that occur within the vasculature must be considered pathologic rather than biologic. It is less clear whether alterations within the vascular media which cause vessels to stiffen should be considered a biologic aging process, or whether these changes, like atherosclerosis, should also be defined as a pathologic entity. While this process does not have an impact on blood flow to organs as is the case for atherosclerosis, it seems to be the cause of an increased systolic blood pressure. This and the resultant mild cardiac hypertrophy and concomitant reduced cardiac filling rate would seem to be the legitimate manifestations of an aging process. The cardiac hypertrophy may be construed as an adaptive mechanism to normalize myocardial wall tension in the presence of increased systolic pressure. The reduced filling rate is physiologically insignificant since cardiac filling volume is not compromised. Clearly, resting cardiac output is not reduced between 20 and 80 years of age.

The imposition of stress such as exercise increases the likelihood of detecting more subtle manifestations of an aging process. Specifically, the prominent age-related change in hemodynamic pattern in response to exercise—a diminished heart rate, enhanced end-systolic volume, and reduced ejection fraction—resembles that observed when the beta-adrenergic system is pharmacologically inhibited. However, adaptive mechanisms like greater end-diastolic filling volume (Starling mechanism) and greater stroke volume can compensate for these deficiencies and thus can prevent a significant decline of cardiac output during exercise in healthy subjects. A higher filling volume, even in the absence of increased myocardial stiffness, would be expected to result in higher filling pressure and therefore a greater tendency for shortness of breath to occur during exercise. It is possible that even this pattern of hemodynamics observed in elderly subjects during exercise, which seems to be attributed to diminished catecholamine responsiveness, may be modified by physical conditioning.

Thus, while certain characteristic age-related changes can be defined in the cardiovascular system, these changes per se do not, at least prior to about 80 years of age, markedly reduce cardiac output, which is the raison d'être of the cardiovascular system. Whether more striking manifestations of an aging process occur in the ninth to eleventh decades in healthy subjects who remain reasonably active and independent community dwellers is currently unknown. When marked declines in cardiac output are observed in elderly subjects between 55 and 80 years of age, causes other than age, such as occult coronary disease or physical deconditioning, must be seriously considered to account for the decline. Our greatest challenge, then, in order to preserve cardiac function in advanced age is not to find a "cure" for biologic aging, but rather to prevent physical deconditioning and especially to understand and conquer atherosclerotic vascular disease. In order to accomplish the latter, investigation must begin in younger age groups, because while this process becomes manifest in middle to late life, it begins much earlier. While epidemiologic methods have implicated an interaction of some life style characteristics and the clinical manifestations of this disease, we are light years away from a true understanding of its pathophysiology. New noninvasive methods which appear to be on the horizon may enable us to begin to detect the vascular lesion prior to onset of its clinical manifestation, at a stage when we can better understand its pathophysiology and more rationally test therapeutic interventions.

NOTES

1. Shock, N. W. Biological theories of aging. In J. R. Florini (ed.), *CRC Handbook of Biochemistry*, pp. 271-282. Boca Raton: CRC Press, 1981.

2. Tejada, C., Strong, J. P., Montenegro, M. R., Restrepo, C., and Solberg, L. A. Distribution of coronary and aortic atherosclerosis by geographic location, race, and sex. *Lab. Invest.* 18:49-66, 1968.

3. Ackerman, R. F., Dry, T. J., and Edwards, J. E. Relationship of various factors to the degree of coronary atherosclerosis in women. *Circulation* 1:1345-1354, 1950.

4. White, N. K., Edwards, J. E., and Dry, T. J. The relationship of the degree of coronary atherosclerosis with age, in men. *Circulation* 1:645-654, 1950.

5. Gerstenblith, G., Fleg, J. L., Vantosh, A., Becker, L., Kallman, C., Andres, R., Weisfeldt, M., and Lakatta, E. G. Stress testing redefines the prevalence of coronary artery disease in epidemiologic studies. *Circulation* 62: Part II, 111-308, 1980.

6. Blumenthal, H. T., Langins, A. I., and Gray, S. H. The interrelation of elastic tissue and calcium in the genesis of arteriosclerosis. *Am. J. Pathol.* 26:989-1009, 1950.

7. Saltin, B., Blomquist, G., Mitchell, J. H., Johnson, R. L., Jr., Wildenthal, K., and Chapman, C. B. Response to exercise after bed rest and after training. A longitudinal study of adaptive changes in oxygen transport and body composition. *Circulation* 38: Suppl 7, VII-1-78, 1968.

8. McGandy, R. B., Barrows, C. H., Jr., Spanias, A., Meredith, A., Stone, J. L., and Norris, A. H. Nutrient intakes and energy expenditure in men of different ages. *J. Gerontol.* 21:581-587, 1966.

9. Rodeheffer, R. J., Gerstenblith, G., Becker, L. C., Fleg, J. L., Weisfeldt, M. L., and Lakatta, E. G. Exercise cardiac output is maintained with advancing age in healthy human subjects: Cardiac dilatation and increased stroke volume compensate for a diminished heart rate. *Circulation* 69:203-213, 1984.

10. Lakatta, E. G. Determinants of cardiovascular performance: Modification due to aging. *J. Chronic Dis.* 36:15-30, 1983.

11. Brandfonbrener, M., Landowne, M., and Shock, N. W. Changes in cardiac output with age. *Circulation* 12:557-566, 1955.

12. Strandell, T. Cardiac output in old age. In F. I. Caird, J. L. C. Dall, and R. D. Kennedy (eds.), *Cardiology in Old Age*, pp. 81-100. New York: Plenum Press, 1976.

13. Gerstenblith, G., Lakatta, E. G., and Weisfeldt, M. L. Age changes in myocardial function and exercise response. *Prog. Cardiovasc. Dis.* 19:1-21, 1976.

14. Kannel, W. B. Blood pressure and the development of cardiovascular disease in the aged. In F. I. Caird, J. L. C. Dall, and R. D. Kennedy (eds.), *Cardiology in Old Age*, pp. 127-175. New York: Plenum Press, 1976.

15. Batsakis, J. G. In S. E. Gould (ed.), *Pathology of the Heart and Blood Vessels*, pp. 519-526. Springfield, Ill.: Charles C Thomas, 3rd ed., 1968.

16. Lakatta, E. G. Alterations in the cardiovascular system that occur in advanced age. *Fed. Proc.* 38:163-167, 1979.

17. Gerstenblith, G., Frederiksen, J., Yin, F. C. P., Fortuin, N. J., Lakatta, E. G., and Weisfeldt, M. L. Echocardiographic assessment of a normal adult aging population. *Circulation* 56:273-278, 1977.

18. Fleg, J. L. Personal communication.

19. Julius, S., Antoon, A., Whitlock, L. S., and Conway, J. Influence of age on the hemodynamic response to exercise. *Circulation* 36:222-230, 1967.

20. Montoye, H. J. *Physical Activity and Health: An Epidemiologic Study of an Entire Community*. Englewood Cliffs, N.J.: Prentice-Hall, 1975.

21. Strandell, T. Circulatory studies on healthy old men. *Acta Med. Scand.* 175: Suppl. 414, 1-44, 1964.

22. Raven, P. B., and Mitchell, J. The effect of aging on the cardiovascular response to dynamic and static exercise. In M. L. Weisfeldt (ed.), *The Aging Heart*, pp. 269-296. New York: Raven Press, 1980.

23. Rerych, S. L., Scholz, P. M., Newman, G. E., Sabiston, D. C., Jr., and Jones, R. H. Cardiac function at rest and during exercise in normals and in patients with coronary heart disease: An evaluation of radionuclide angiocardiography. *Ann. Surg.* 187:449-464, 1978.

24. Port, E., Cobb, F. R., Coleman, R. E., and Jones, R. H. Effect of age on the response of the left ventricular ejection fraction to exercise. *New Engl. J. Med.* 303:1133-1137, 1980.

25. Yin, F. C. P., Weisfeldt, M. L., and Milnor, W. R. Role of aortic input impedance in the decreased cardiovascular response to exercise with aging in dogs. *J. Clin. Invest.* 68:28-38, 1981.

26. Tzankoff, S. T., Fleg, J. L., Norris, A. H., and Lakatta, E. G. Age-related increase in serum catecholamine levels during exercise in healthy adult men. *Physiologist* 23:50, 1980.

27. Lakatta, E. G. Age-related alterations in the cardiovascular response to adrenergic mediated stress. *Fed. Proc.* 39:3173-3177, 1980.

28. Conway, J., Wheeler, R., and Sannerstedt, R. Sympathetic nervous activity during exercise in relation to age. *Cardiovasc. Res.* 5:577-581, 1971.

29. Yin, F. C. P., Spurgeon, H. A., Raizes, G. S., Greene, H. L., Weisfeldt, M. L., and Shock, N. W. Age-associated decrease in heart rate response to isoproterenol in dogs. *Circulation* 54: Suppl. 2, 11-167, 1976.

30. Yin, F. C. P., Spurgeon, H. A., Raizes, G. S., Greene, H. L., Weisfeldt, M. L., and Shock, N. W. Age-associated decrease in heart rate response to isoproterenol in dogs. *Mech. Aging Dev.* 10:17-25, 1979.

31. Fleisch, J. H., and Hooker, C. S. The relationship between age and relaxation of vascular smooth muscle in the rabbit and rat. *Circ. Res.* 38:243-249, 1976.

32. Filburn, C. R., and Lakatta, E. G. Aging alterations in β-adrenergic modulation of cardiac cell function. In J. Johnson, Jr. (ed.), *Aging and Cell Function,* Volume 2, pp. 211-246. New York: Plenum Press, 1984.

33. Guarnieri, T., Filburn, C. R., Zitnik, G., Roth, G. S., and Lakatta, E. G. Contractile and biochemical correlates of β-adrenergic stimulation of the aged heart. *Am. J. Physiol.* 239:H501-H508, 1980.

34. Lakatta, E. G., Gerstenblith, G., Angell, C. S., Shock, N. W., and Weisfeldt, M. L. Diminished inotropic response of aged myocardium to catecholamines. *Circ. Res.* 36:262-269, 1975.

Depressive Illness in Late Life

Dan Blazer*

Simone de Beauvoir (1970) tells of the young Buddha, Prince Siddhartha, who frequently would ride into the countryside from his beautiful palace. On one of the first visits away, he saw a tottering, wrinkled, white-haired decrepit old man who was bent over, trembling, and mumbling something almost incomprehensible while he slowly progressed on his journey with the aid of a walking stick. The young prince was astonished and frightened and told his charioteer, "It is the world's pity, that weak and ignorant beings, drunk with the vanity of youth, do not behold old age. Let us hurry back to the palace. What is the use of pleasures in the life, since I myself am the future dwelling-place of old age?" As with the young prince, themes of age and depression often coexist. In fact, discouragement, hopelessness, and helplessness are often considered synonymous with the aging process.

Those who have seriously observed older persons through time, however, are well aware that most of them are satisfied with their lives and undergo only minor fluctuations in their moods (Palmore and Kivett, 1970). In fact, older persons may have considerable prestige, financial security, and freedom to engage in

*Associate Professor of Psychiatry; Head, Division of Social and Community Psychiatry; and Senior Fellow, Center for the Study of Aging and Human Development, Duke University Medical Center, Durham, North Carolina.

many useful and enjoyable activities not available at earlier stages of the life cycle. Therefore, "depression" must not be assumed to coalesce with the process of aging. Nevertheless, depressive illness, which may contribute to significantly decreased functioning in older persons and may even be life-threatening, is a relatively frequent illness in late life when compared with other public health concerns. Rather than enter a long-standing and well-documented defense of the general life satisfaction among older adults, or comment on the discouragement and dissatisfaction among older persons which derive from societal ills, I will limit this discussion to the more severe episodes of depression which occur among the elderly. My basic premise is that depressive illness is a not uncommon, severe, but potentially treatable health problem in late life. The conceptual framework of modern medicine, which has contributed greatly to our understanding of many illnesses including senile dementia, hypertension, and cancer, may be applied to the study of depressive illness as well.

WHAT IS DEPRESSIVE ILLNESS?

Clinicians who treat older patients with emotional illnesses must focus their diagnostic skills on the thoughts, feelings, and actions of the person being examined, in contrast to the diagnosis of most physical illnesses (Linn, 1975). Symptoms and signs of depression among the elderly are determined not only by reports and observable evidence of distress in the individual, but also by observations that the individual's interaction with the social environment is disturbed. If depressive symptoms and depressive illness are unchanged through the life cycle, then those traditional approaches to diagnosis would require no modification in late life. Yet depressive illness may appear in a unique way among the elderly.

The elderly may be thought of as a group of individuals who have been exposed to a different culture from persons at earlier stages of the life cycle, i.e., the present "cohort" of older persons has experienced a series of historical events at critical stages of their development which are quite different from the events experienced by other age cohorts. For example, the elderly, during their childhood, experienced child-rearing practices that were devoid of our present knowledge of the Freudian stages of child development, not to mention the absence of the influence of Dr.

Spock's *Baby and Child Care*. Psychological awareness and insight were de-emphasized during these critical developmental transitions, whereas regularity and discipline in certain areas, such as toilet training, were emphasized. It should therefore not surprise one to find that older persons tend to understand their feelings of discomfort more in terms of physical discomfort than psychological or emotional discomfort. This "cohort effect" has thus led many investigators to suggest that our present approaches to the diagnosis of depressive illness, developed primarily from work with persons in early and mid-life, are not applicable to older persons; these approaches are reviewed below (Blazer, 1980).

Depressive symptoms are characteristic of a number of human conditions, some of which qualify as depressive illness and some of which do not. The most common situation contributing to depressive symptoms is bereavement, a universal human experience and the normal response to the loss of a loved one, job, economic security, or even one's dwelling unit. Closely associated with bereavement is the emotional adjustment of older persons to stressful events in their lives, such as a move to a retirement community or the development of a potentially fatal or chronically debilitating illness. Loss of the ability to function physically and socially, not to mention anticipation of the termination of life, will usually precipitate symptoms of depression.

A nonspecific distress conceptualized as "demoralization" (Frank, 1979) has been identified as a not infrequent symptom complex in community populations. Demoralization is characteristic for most persons seeking "help" regardless of whether they are suffering from a psychiatric disorder or not, and occurs when a person "finds that he cannot meet the demands placed on him by the environment, and cannot extricate himself from his predicament." According to Dohrenwend and his colleagues (1980), the nonspecific distress of demoralization is reflected by a series of symptoms, including poor self-esteem, helplessness–hopelessness, dread, sadness, anxiety, confused thinking, psychophysiologic symptoms, and perceived poor health. Dissatisfaction with one's life and existential anxiety may also contribute to this particular symptom complex. None of the above, however, can truly be labeled "depressive illness," but one must not minimize the suffering experienced by persons with these symptoms. The cause of such symptoms can usually be traced to physical illness, unresolved interpersonal relationships, or difficult problems of living.

In contrast, depressive illness is of more severe proportions, of longer duration, and cannot be easily traced to and explained by circumstances encountered by the individual suffering from such an episode. Depressive illness has recently been defined as a "major depressive episode" by the American Psychiatric Association (1980), with persons required to meet certain symptom criteria to be so diagnosed. These episodes are characterized by a dysphoric mood or loss of interest or pleasure in all or almost all usual activities and pastimes. Accompanying symptoms such as the expression of depression, sadness, hopelessness, being "down in the dumps," and irritability are the "criteria symptoms" which must be present nearly every day for a period of at least 2 weeks. The individual must demonstrate at least four of these symptoms to qualify for a diagnosis of a major depressive episode. These symptoms include poor appetite or weight loss, sleep disturbances, loss of energy, agitation or retardation in movement, loss of interest or pleasure in usual activities or decrease in sexual drive, feelings of self-reproach or excessive and inappropriate guilt, complaints or evidence of diminished ability to think or concentrate, and recurrent thoughts of death or suicidal ideation. The episodes of depressive illness typically do not extend indefinitely, but may persist for as long as 2 years.

More severe, gross impairments in reality testing may occur, suggesting a psychiatric process, though the condition must be distinguished from schizophrenia. A biologically driven depression is suggested when the individual experiences the depression more severely in the morning, tends to awaken early in the morning, exhibits marked motor retardation or agitation, experiences significant loss of appetite and weight, and expresses excessive and inappropriate feelings of guilt. These persons, regardless of the etiology of their depressive symptoms, do not respond well to psychosocial intervention and have been labeled as having "autonomous" depression (Friedel, 1983). Much less frequently, symptoms of depressive illness may be preceded or succeeded by symptoms of mania or hypomania (elation, exaggerated self-esteem, and exuberant happiness). Speech in the manic patient is often circumstantial and obsessive, and the patient is frequently agitated (though the overactivity is not as pronounced as in manic episodes appearing earlier in life). Paranoid delusions are frequently seen in the manic elder.

In recent years, clinicians have identified still another category of individuals who suffer from depressive symptoms but who do not easily fit into the diagnoses described above. These persons are suffering from, for want of a better term, atypical depression (Quitkin et al., 1979). Atypical depressions are uniquely responsive to pharmacological therapies, especially to drugs from the class of monoamine oxidase inhibitors; a precipitating factor is common; and the mild and often variable depression is often masked by anxiety, somatic complaints, and histrionic behavior. Such individuals tend to exhibit hypersomnia and hyperphagia, in contrast to the sleep difficulties and loss of appetite usually seen in depressive illness.

Other psychiatric disorders in older persons may be confused with depressive illness. By far the most common are the dementias. Senile dementia of the Alzheimer's type and Parkinson's disease may lead to significant depressive symptoms early in their course and, given the memory impairment and withdrawal from the social environment that sometimes occur, may suggest depressive illness. It is more common, however, for depressive symptoms in the elderly to appear to a clinician as a dementia, leading to the use of the term "pseudodementia." Nevertheless, early dementias may be overlooked in favor of a diagnosis of depressive illness. Hypochondriasis, an exaggerated concern about the body that is a not uncommon problem in the elderly, may also be confused with depression. In contrast to the definite and usually datable onset of depression, hypochondriasis develops gradually and both patient and family have difficulty in assigning a particular time period to the start of the perceived problems. Sleep problems and subsequent concern about the disruption of normal sleep that is usual in late life may also be interpreted as a depressive disorder when in fact the sleep disturbance itself is the primary problem. Finally, intoxication with medications, usually those prescribed by physicians, frequently leads to depressive symptoms in older persons. Offenders among the more commonly prescribed drugs include reserpine, beta-blockers such as propranolol (Inderal), cortisol, antianxiety and sedative–hypnotic agents such as diazepam (Valium), flurazepam (Dalmane), and the barbiturates.

Many questions still confront researchers and clinicians who attempt to categorize older persons suffering from depressive symptoms. Do the arbitrary distinctions made between the different categories described above reflect reality? Undoubtedly overlap exists, but is that overlap so extensive that the present categories are virtually useless for predicting a particular outcome or a response to a particular type of treatment? How reliably can we delineate the differences between these categories? Even if we set up what appear to be rather exacting criteria for categorizing individuals, are clinicians and researchers capable of consistently classifying individuals accordingly? Finally, if many depressive symptoms among older persons can be explained primarily on the basis of environmental circumstances, such as bereavement or demoralization, what is the role of the health care profession in providing assistance to these individuals?

THE BURDEN OF DEPRESSION IN THE ELDERLY

The study of late-life depression cannot be limited to the clinician's office or the laboratory. To appreciate the nature and extent of depression in populations and through time, the methods of epidemiology have been employed in helping to answer some of the following questions relevant to the burden of depression in the elderly (Morris, 1975):

• What is the rate of depressive illness among the elderly and how does this rate vary with sex, race, or socioeconomic status?

• Have the rates of depression among the elderly changed over time?

• Do older adults with major depressive illness seek professional help?

• What type of health services are provided to the depressed elderly?

• To what degree are older persons functionally impaired because of their depressive symptoms?

Measures of disease frequency, stated in terms permitting comparisons between populations, are the foundation of epidemiology (MacMahon and Pugh, 1979). To allow for differences in population size or for comparisons within populations, frequencies are expressed as rates—the frequency of a disease or characteristic per unit of the population or group being observed. The rates of depressive symptoms and depressive illness in community, clinic, and inpatient populations are presented from representative studies in Table 1.

As can be seen, depending on the approach to identification of individuals suffering from depression, rates will vary. If one con-

TABLE 1 Rates of Depressive Symptoms and Depressive Illness in Community, Clinic, and Inpatient Populations

Population	Depressive Illness Rate (%)	Author
Community sample of New Haven, Conn.	5.4	Weissman and Myers (1978)
Psychogeriatric outpatients in Lausanne, Switzerland	19.0	Wertheimer et al. (1973)
Psychogeriatric inpatient unit	19.0	Daniel (1972)
	Depressive Symptom Rate (%)	
Community sample of Durham County, N.C.	14.7	Blazer and Williams (1980)
Geriatric clinic	33.0	Blazer (1978a)
Geriatric ward	31.3	Cheach and Beard (1980)

siders only significant depressive symptoms, which may be associated with normal grief or a reaction to physical illness, the rates are much higher, reaching 15 percent in the community. In contrast, if one uses specific criteria for making a diagnosis of depressive illness (as described above), the rates are closer to 5 percent. These rates increase when outpatient and inpatient populations are considered. Most researchers who have studied community populations report that depressive symptoms increase with age. In contrast, there is no evidence that major depressive disorders increase with age, and in fact, the rates may be somewhat lower among the elderly than they are in persons in the middle of the life cycle (Weissman and Myers, 1978). According to more recent studies, females continue to have a proportionately increased rate of depression when compared to males in late life, as they do at other stages of the life cycle (Myers et al., 1982).

Unfortunately, these rates alone do not accurately reflect the burden of late life depression in our society. For example, suicide rates increase almost linearly with age, an increase explained predominately by an age-related increase in suicide rates among white males (U.S. Department of Health, Education and Welfare, 1978). Although there is widespread concern about the rate of suicide among adolescents, a tragic and frequently publicized event, the rate of suicide among those 85 and older is almost four times as great. In addition, overall dysfunction resulting from depression in the elderly is significant. For example, 28 percent of those suffering from a major depressive illness were found to be suffering from an impairment in social functioning, and 28 percent were economically impaired (Blazer and Williams, 1980).

The depressed elderly, as is true of individuals at all stages of the life cycle, tend to use primary care physicians as their principal source of care (Regier, 1978; Blazer and Williams, 1980). The use of psychiatric services by the elderly is much lower than use by persons at other stages of the life cycle: less than 1 percent of the older community population seek or are actively engaged in counseling or other psychiatric and psychological services (Blazer and Williams, 1980). In contrast, older persons more frequently use psychotherapeutic medications. The benzodiazepines, which include drugs like diazepam (Valium) and chlordiazepoxide (Librium), are among the most commonly prescribed medications in this country for all age groups, and are more frequently prescribed for older persons than for any other age group (Balter et al., 1974). In one study, the phenothiazine class of drugs was the most frequently prescribed class in a nursing home population, outranking even the prescription of drugs to treat the cardiovascular system (Ray et al., 1980). As documented by Ray et al. (1980), there is reason to believe that these medications are often overprescribed or misprescribed. For example, the frequency with which the symptom of depression occurs would lead one to assume that antidepressant medications are widely used in this population. Nevertheless, they are not among the more commonly prescribed drugs, and therefore it must be questioned whether these generally effective medications are being adequately used in the elderly for major depressive illness.

Though information from epidemiologic studies of depression in the elderly and the use of various methods of health care by those suffering from depression have increased in recent years, many questions remain unanswered. For example, are the elderly who seek treatment for major depressive illnesses different from those who are untreated? Why do elderly white males continue to commit suicide at a significantly higher rate than any other demographic group? Are major depressive illnesses in late life qualitatively different from such illnesses occuring at other stages of the life cycle, e.g., do the episodes last longer or are the elderly more subject to recurrences of their illness? What factors prevent older adults from receiving adequate treatment for their depressive disorders?

THE ORIGINS OF LATE-LIFE DEPRESSION

States of health, not to mention illness, are understood fully only in terms of their biological, psychological, and social parameters, and health care as well as research must be correspondingly oriented (Reiser, 1980). Persons suffering from depressive symptomatology in late life can be regarded as living systems, composed of subsystems that form part of a larger environmental suprasystem—the "whole" being an open system which allows free transactional interactions of energy and information across system boundaries. This concept serves as the foundation of the biopsychosocial model for understanding late-life depressive illness. The brain is a subsystem regulated by homoscedastic mechanisms geared to maintain an adaptive internal environment in the face of external environmental challenges. In psychology, the "mind" comprises the psychological subsystem of the person who articulates and interacts with the meanings (e.g., symbols) found in the environment. From the perspective of the social sciences, "persons" are parts of social groups and therefore are influenced by other members of these groups.

Late-life depressive illness provides researchers as well as clinicians with an opportunity to conceptualize a relatively common malady effectively in terms of this multidimensional model. Though no evidence to date suggests that older persons are more likely to encounter depressive illness, certain biological, psychological, and social factors may uniquely predispose some older persons to serious episodes of depression, these are illustrated below. Not one of these potential contributing factors is either necessary or sufficient for the onset of late-life depression. Rather, the "genealogy" of late-life depression may best be thought of as a web which, in its complexity and origins, lies quite beyond our total understanding (MacMahon and Pugh, 1979). Figure 1 illustrates some of the nodal points within this web of causation.

The biological origins of late-life depression have generally been separated into four potential categories. First, following a major thrust in the biological research of affective disorders, are those studies focusing on neurotransmitter abnormalities. Neurotransmitters are those chemical substances which transfer in-

114

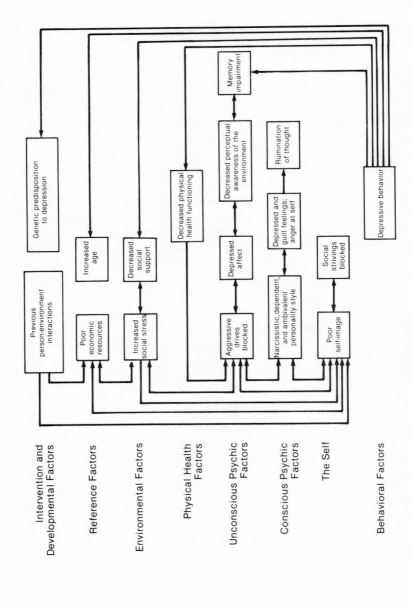

FIGURE 1 Some components in the etiology of depression in late life. Reprinted, with permission, from Blazer, D. G. "Epidemiology of Mental Illness in Late Life." In Busse, E. W., and Blazer, D. G., eds., *Handbook of Geriatric Psychiatry.* New York: Van Nostrand Reinhold, 1980, p. 262.

formation from one neuron to another across the synapse, the gap between neurons. For example, the "catecholamine hypothesis" of depressive illness states that a depletion of brain catecholamines (especially norepinephrine) as well as of the indoleamines (especially serotonin) precipitates episodes of depressive illness (Schildkraut, 1965). The medications that have been found most effective in treating late-life depression are known to increase the level of catecholamines in the brain (Mendels et al., 1976). Samorajski and his colleagues (1971) have found that whole-brain levels of norepinephrine, serotonin, and acetylcholine decrease significantly with age, suggesting that the catecholamine system is most vulnerable to the process of aging.

Second, recent attention has been increasingly directed to endocrine disturbances in the depressed. For example, it has long been known that a significant number of depressed patients hypersecrete cortisol and that persons challenged with dexamethasone, a synthetic steroid, do not demonstrate the normal regulatory decrease in the production of cortisol seen in nondepressed adults. This finding is illustrated more thoroughly below in the discussion of the dexamethasone suppression test. In addition, other researchers have demonstrated that thyroid function may be adversely affected in the depressed. Although pituitary thyroid stimulating hormone (TSH) secretion is generally within normal limits, it is under the control of a hypothymic hormone, thyrotropin releasing hormone (TRH). The usual elevation of TSH following administration of TRH has been shown to be blunted in the elderly (Loosen et al., 1977). Aging definitely leads to changes in the neuroendocrine system. For example, studies in humans and animals suggest a decline in the responsiveness of the adrenal cortex to adrenocorticotropic hormone (ACTH) with aging (Bowman and Wolf, 1969), though there is no convincing evidence that this significantly alters the response of the pituitary gland to the exogenous steroid dexamethasone. Studies in humans substantiate previous animal research which reports a significant decrease in the magnitude of TRH-induced TSH response. Therefore, the endocrine changes normally observed in the depressed may be complicated by the aging process, not to mention the frequent illnesses accompanying late life (such as heart disease and diabetes mellitus) that may significantly contribute to endocrine abnormalities.

Of great interest, as described below, is the potential for a more accurate diagnosis of depressive illness through an examination of the sleep architecture of depressed subjects when compared to that of normal subjects. Unfortunately, sleep architecture in aging changes significantly, and these changes are often in the direction of the abnormalities identified with depression, namely, decreased sleep efficiency, intermittent wakefulness, decreased deep sleep, and especially a decline in rapid eye movement (REM) sleep latency. As demonstrated below, age-adjusted normal sleep variables can be developed and used effectively for clinical diagnosis in the sleep laboratory despite these age-related changes (Kupfer et al., 1982).

Finally, there is considerable evidence, especially from twin and family studies (Slater and Cowie, 1971), of a genetic contribution to the etiology of depression. Yet preliminary research suggests that the genetic contribution to depressive disorders in late life is weaker than at other stages of the life cycle (Hopkinson, 1964; Mendlewicz, 1976). Unfortunately, family data collected for older persons is less reliable because of subjects' declining memory and the death or geographic separation of relatives. Nevertheless, the influence of genetically determined factors presumably begins before late life as environmental pressures accumulate with time, suggesting that depressive illness in later life may be a condition caused by such pressures and declining physical functioning.

The psychoanalytic literature is replete with explanations of why the older person should be psychologically predisposed to the development of depressive symptoms. Yet these theories must be considered within the context that most older persons are quite satisfied with their status in life, and that the prevalence of serious depressive illness is no more a problem in late life than at earlier stages of the life cycle. Nevertheless, some of these theories can be instructive. Eric Erikson (1950) was one of the first to develop a theory of personality development that specifically included adulthood and aging as well as childhood and adolescence. The last stage of his eight-stage representation of crisis and adaptation is the development of a sense of ego integrity, namely, the conscious assurance of order and meaning in life. The absence of this developmental milestone is manifested by despair—the feeling that remaining life is short, "too short for the attempt to start another life and to try alternate roads to integrity." Wigdor (1980) expands this theme by noting that in our achievement-oriented society, the major reinforcers lead to the development of habit patterns and emphasize incentives for activity that may not be adaptive or appropriate to the changing life patterns occurring with advanced age. Lazarus and Weinberg (1980), on the other hand, emphasize the potential for injury to self-concept, i.e., narcissistic injury. Such perceived slights in older adults may manifest themselves in "recurring depressions or defensive grandiosity, self consciousness, overdependence and approval from others for maintenance of self esteem, and the transitory periods of fragmentation and discohesiveness of the self." Kath (1965) believes that the desire to restore functioning secondary to the inevitable losses in late life is a major developmental task of aging individuals. Yet at a conscious level the older adult recognizes a decline in the drives and instincts usually experienced early in life. A coexisting decline in demands from the outside for achievement may necessitate a denunciation of previous activities toward development of formal relationships and successful completion of tasks. Therefore, if one lives sufficiently long, the inevitable loss of friends and loved ones, body changes, and disease lead to a state of internal and external depletion which in turn may be associated with the uncomfortable state of apparent emotional exile and impending death.

Despite the predominant emphasis on psychoanalytic theories of depression in late life, contributions have also come from both the proponents of learning theory and those individuals who have looked at specific psychological processes such as motivation. "Learned helplessness" (Seligman, 1974) is perhaps the best known behavioral model of depression. Because of inescapable adverse stimuli, animals were noted in laboratory experiments to "give up" and passively accept the stimuli, the behavioral symptoms of learned helplessness being failure to initiate responses and difficulty in learning that a new response might be effective in alleviating a painful situation even when one is presented. Older persons may be at greater risk than individuals at other stages of the life cycle for being placed in situations in which their own behavior apparently has little effect on the behavior of other persons. This is especially true when physical health or cognitive functioning has been inaccurately assessed or when treatment interventions have been prescribed which are restrictive and preclude consultation with the older person.

Motivation, comprising those energizers of behavior in general and the sources of energy in particular situations which keep a person's behavior goal-directed, is a major contributor to the continuity and persistence of certain behaviors. Researchers have examined evidence of "slowing" of the central nervous system with aging, and suggest that the amount of stimulation needed for arousal is probably higher for the elderly (Wigdor, 1980). For example, there is evidence of some reduction in drive related to food and drink consumption with aging, while there is little evidence to suggest that the psychological needs for food and drink decrease significantly. Since a decline in motivation consistently accompanies depressive illness, the interaction of normal changes in motivation with aging and changes associated with depression must be distinguished if one is truly to understand the origins of depression.

Loss and response to loss of persons important to an older individual's social environment have for many years been hypothesized as being the primary contributor to late-life depression (Freud, 1917). Interest in the relationship of the social environment to the onset and outcome of physical as well as psychiatric illness has blossomed during the past 15 years (Cassel, 1976; MacMahon and Pugh, 1979). The elderly have traditionally been assumed to be at greater risk for stressful life events. For example, Butler (1974) lists a series of predictable stressful events in late life, such as attempts to force older persons into preconceived cultural definitions as dependent, roleless, and incompetent. "Ageism" expresses this prejudice toward older persons. Loss of status and prestige occurs as social roles are lost parallel to the loss of employment and economic status. Financial problems are thought to be common in late life. Older persons are also at greater risk for the loss of spouse, siblings, friends, and even children. Yet Neugarten (1970), while noting that older persons do encounter a higher frequency of certain stressful events, suggests that they may be better prepared to accept and adapt to these experiences than persons at earlier stages of the life cycle. Most older persons anticipate certain events, such as the loss of loved ones. Unanticipated events are much more likely to be traumatic. Yet older persons do experience unique stressful events that may be particularly disruptive, especially to the social relationship. Many studies suggest that older persons are at greater risk for impaired social relations and support (Lowenthal and Berkman, 1967). Older persons may become socially isolated, many times by choice. Whether voluntary or not, this isolation limits their ability to participate in social and healthful activities. Geographic isolation may lead to decreased ties with family. Studies have demonstrated that a deficient social network is associated with increased depressive symptomatology (Blazer, 1983).

It is doubtful that, given the nature of depressive illness in late life, a unitary theory of depressive illness will be forthcoming. It is always tempting to retreat to such a theory, because the implications are that intervention at one point, for instance, by administering a particular medication or readjusting some identified environmental stressor, would immediately and predictably correct the problem. Yet experience with the spectrum of depressive illness in the elderly leads one to discount a unitary theory of depressive etiology. At best, we can identify potential risk factors—i.e., factors frequently associated with depressive disorders both in cross-sectional and longitudinal studies—and identify their relative strength. Though no single factor may persistently be the culprit, a constellation of factors given variable weights, leading to an algorithm, could prove invaluable to clinicians assessing the etiology of depressive symptomatology in the elderly. Future research should be directed to solidifying our understanding of the individual risk factors, their reliable identification, and the correct assignment of relative risks for each.

DIAGNOSTIC WORK-UP OF THE PATIENT WITH DEPRESSION

The cornerstone of the diagnostic work-up of the depressed older adult, regardless of the suspected etiology, is a thorough history from the patient and a family member. No laboratory tests can replace the perspective of history on depressive symptoms within the context of an individual's life, i.e., a thorough understanding of depressive symptoms, the circumstances of their onset, methods by which the individual has attempted to adapt to these symptoms, and subsequent problems in social functioning. Accompanying the history is the "mental status examination," the systematic appraisal of the patient's emotional and cognitive functioning. Though mood can usually be determined by observing the patient during the interview process, specific questions must be addressed to the patient to assess certain abilities to reason, remember, and solve novel problems. Well-trained clinicians are able, during the course of the interview, to accurately assess the prevalent mood of the patient and whether this mood is congruent with the experiences the patient describes. As older patients are frequently less communicative and articulate than younger ones in describing their depressive moods, an awareness of the variety of demeanors that a depressed older person may present to the clinician is invaluable, as are techniques for effectively communicating with the elderly depressed patient (Blazer, 1978b).

Only a few years ago, the history and mental status examination provided the only means by which clinicians were capable of diagnosing depressive disorders in any age group. Recently, a number of diagnostic laboratory tests have been developed to identify "biological markers" of depressive illness. The best known and most extensively used test at present is the dexamethasone suppression test (Carroll et al., 1981). Patients suffering from depressive illness frequently do not shut down the pituitary production of ACTH following the introduction of the synthetic steroid dexamethasone. This is in sharp contrast to the usual well-adapted regulatory mechanisms in normal persons throughout the life cycle. Evidence to date suggests that the dexamethasone suppression test can be useful in identifying older persons suffering from depressive illness and may in fact be of benefit in predicting a future response to drug treatments. Unfortunately, the test result may be abnormal in persons suffering from one of the dementias, especially a dementia in the more severe stages (Raskind et al., 1982). Depressed patients have also been found to have a similar "blunted response" in the release of another pituitary hormone, TSH, in response to the administration of protyrelin, a synthetic TRH. Some patients with depressive illness have a normal dexamethasone suppression test but an abnormal TSH response to TRH. Therefore, the TSH stimulation test may be especially useful in older persons with clinical features suggesting depressive illness, but who have a normal response to the dexamethasone test (Loosen and Prange, 1982).

Sleep studies are not nearly as easily performed as the laboratory studies described above. Nevertheless, a change in sleep in the depressed has been documented consistently in the literature (Kupfer et al., 1982). Specifically, there is a persistent decline in REM sleep latency (the time from sleep onset to the first period of REM sleep) among the depressed. Unfortunately, the normal changes in the sleep cycle that occur with age tend to interfere with potential diagnostic tests for depressive illness in the elderly. Nevertheless, Kupfer and colleagues (1982) have developed a series of age-corrected sleep variables that can be used to distinguish the normal changes in sleep with aging from those changes that may occur secondary to depressive illness. By using such age-corrected values, 65 percent of a group of depressed older persons were found to demonstrate REM latency while only 5 percent of those not depressed demonstrated the same finding.

The advent of these diagnostic tests has literally opened a new era to clinicians in the continued search for more effective means of distinguishing persons with depressive illness. Questions do remain, however. To what degree do normal age-related changes in endocrine function, sleep, etc., interfere with the predictability and value of these increasingly widely used diagnostic tests? Do the biological changes occurring with depression in some way overlap the changes that occur with dementia and therefore decrease the potential value of these tests in older persons with multiple problems? Will these tests be as valuable in predicting responses to drug treatments in older persons, especially given the potential for adverse side effects in the elderly, as they are at earlier stages of the life cycle?

TREATMENT OF LATE-LIFE DEPRESSION

The treatment of depression throughout the life cycle entails the use of both biological and nonbiological interventions. Given the etiological model described above, it is self-evident that rarely will a single treatment approach in isolation be sufficient to treat true depressive illness. In fact, it is difficult for a clinician to work "in isolation," for the physician prescribing medications must effectively communicate with and support the older adult (a form of psychotherapy), whereas the psychotherapist cannot ignore the realities of the social environment in which the depressed elder is situated.

Many advances in the pharmacologic treatment of depressive illness are derived from the catecholamine hypothesis of depressive illness described above. The tricyclic antidepressants, a class of drugs including amitriptyline (Elavil), doxepin (Sinequan), and nortriptyline (Aventyl, Pamelor), have been the first line pharmacologic treatment of depressive disorders in adults and elders since their discovery in the late 1950s. Though the neuropharmacologic effects of these drugs continue to be investigated, their ability to increase norepinephrine and serotonin in key areas of the brain (within the synaptic cleft) undoubtedly is closely associated with their effectiveness. Unfortunately, older persons tolerate the tricyclic antidepressants poorly. Though cardiac problems, such as arrhythmias, are the most serious side effects, "anticholinergic effects" such as dryness of the mouth, constipation, blurring of vision, confusion, and postural hypotension are the most frequent and disturbing of the side effects (Nies et al., 1977).

Because of the problems with side effects from these frequently prescribed medications, other drugs with fewer side effects have been prescribed for depressive symptoms in late life, some with good justification and some without. For example, methylphenidate (Ritalin), a stimulant which has a similar pharmacological action to the amphetamines, has been used frequently, especially in nursing home populations. There is a potential, at least in theory, for both addiction and serious problems with overdose, but when used in relatively low doses this drug causes few side effects and appears to be well tolerated by many older adults. It is not a true antidepressant and has been documented in very few studies to be of value to older persons, but nevertheless continues to be used (Crook, 1979). Hydergine, a dihydroergot alkaloid recommended primarily for the treatment of dementia, is also thought to be a mild stimulant with relatively few side effects; it may in fact improve functioning in dementia patients by means of its potential for general activation and its mild antidepressant effect. The drug has proved effective in a number of controlled studies (Cole, 1980). Prange et al. (1970) reported that the addition of low doses of triiodothyronine to the tricyclic antidepressants potentiates the therapeutic response to these agents, especially in women. Though thyroid has not been used extensively in older depressed patients, these findings may have implications for the elderly, as thyroid gland function does change with age, which in turn may indirectly affect the catecholamine system.

Of great interest to clinicians working with older persons has been the advent of a new generation of antidepressant agents, most of which do not contain the basic tricyclic chemical structure of the well-known antidepressant agents. There is little evidence to date that these agents are sufficiently better antidepressants with appreciably fewer side effects than earlier antidepressant drugs to warrant a major redirection in our therapeutic approach to older adults. Nevertheless, these drugs may give clinicians more flexibility in treating older depressed patients. For example, as mentioned above, anticholinergic effects are among the most disturbing the clinician faces in treating older depressed adults. Trazodone (Desyrel) is a new-generation antidepressant with virtually no anticholinergic effects. Though it is not without side effects (it can be quite sedating), it may be uniquely suited for treating certain agitated depressed older adults who are particularly sensitive to the anticholinergic effects of the tricyclic drugs.

Electroconvulsive therapy (ECT), despite the negative reaction that often accompanies the mention of "electroshock," is a valuable treatment option for depressed older adults. In severe depressive illness with psychotic symptomatology resistant to medications, ECT frequently is the only treatment that is effective (Weiner, 1982). Unique and age-specific techniques for administering ECT to older adults, such as unilateral electrode placement, have improved the efficacy and safety of this treatment to the point where it is safer and frequently more effective than medications. Two problems persist, however. First, the societal view of ECT appropriately relegates the treatment to situations where other modes of therapy have failed. Second, the usual but transient memory loss that accompanies a course of ECT can be especially disturbing to older persons with "pseudodementia," namely, those individuals who already complain of memory loss as the central symptom of their depressive illness.

Psychotherapy for the depressed older adult has received scant attention in the literature relative to its potential for benefit and the frequency of its use. Recent work by a number of therapists (Steuer, 1982) suggests that short-term cognitive-behavioral therapy may be specific for depressive symptoms and especially suitable to older adults. Beck et al. (1979) claimed that cognitive-behavior therapy differs from more traditional therapies in the high activity level of the therapist, the focus on present-day problems, and the constant emphasis on reality testing and tasks assigned to the patient between sessions. Most clinicians recognize the necessity of involving family members in the therapy process as well (Blazer, 1982a). Not only must the clinician thoroughly evaluate the family, but family members should be alerted to the symptoms of worsening depression and taught the nature of depressive illness in late life. Families must recognize the potential outcome risks of depression in late life, such as suicide. Preliminary work with families can often alleviate considerable guilt when this infrequent but tragic event occurs.

Finally, clinicians working with older adults recognize that the severely depressed frequently must be hospitalized. Psychiatric facilities traditionally have not been designed to care for the elderly, but the increasing numbers of older adults using these facilities have led to the creation of geriatric psychiatry units that specialize in the care of older persons. Given the risk for suicide and the burden of depressive symptoms upon family members, hospitalization of the depressed patient should not be postponed or neglected. Unfortunately, the reduction in benefits for the mentally ill elderly may, in the future, limit our ability to treat the depressed older adult with these tested and proven methods of therapy.

Many questions remain unanswered by clinicians and researchers devoted to treating depressed older adults. Though the majority of older adults respond well to the treatment of depressive illness, a small but significant percentage do not respond. This is especially disturbing when one considers the remarkable advances in the pharmacologic therapy of depression, almost to the point that many clinicians will virtually "guarantee" success with a given pharmacologic agent. The persistent problem with respect to antidepressant medications is their side effects. What drugs at what dose levels are therapeutic but relatively free of disturbing side effects? What methods can be employed to increase the compliance of patients in completing a clinical course of antidepressant medication when side effects present a problem? As at other stages of the life cycle, to date no one has determined why antidepressant medications require 2 to 3 weeks before a therapeutic response occurs.

New horizons in our understanding of late-life depression, especially disturbances in circadian rhythms, may provide increased insight into the etiology of such depression, not to mention an ultimate "pay-off" in the management of these patients. For example, are there methods of adjusting the sleep cycle that will improve the efficacy of our treatment of late-life depression? Can certain activities be prescribed to older adults at certain times during the day, or can diets be adjusted in such a way that symptoms can be alleviated?

Finally, we must persist in documenting the effectiveness of various innovative treatments of late-life depression. Scarcity of resources will necessarily limit the availability of the broad range of potential therapies available for the depressed older adult. Which of these therapies, if one must choose from among them, are most effective for which patients? No simple or inevitably accurate "decision trees" are likely to be forthcoming; nevertheless clinicians can, with accurate methodology and follow-up, make important progress in choosing therapies and evaluating their results.

Our persistence in attempting to understand the epidemiology, etiology, and biological, psychological, and social characteristics of depressive illness will continue to push the field forward. Nevertheless, the patient must not be forgotten, for if the older person suffering from depressive illness does not perceive his or her problems within the same context that we view the disease process, our interactions with these persons will prove unproductive. Communication with those suffering from late life depressive illness not only increases our knowledge, but also our empathy. Empathy, in turn, is essential in communicating to the depressed elder our desire to help and our potential as care providers to form a therapeutic alliance in the service of their improved psychiatric health.

REFERENCES AND BIBLIOGRAPHY

American Psychiatric Association. *Diagnostic and Statistical Manual of Mental Disorders* (3rd Ed.). Washington, D.C., 1980.

Balter, M., et al. "Cross-National Study of the Extent of Antianxiety and Sedative Drug Use." *New England Journal of Medicine* 290:769, 1974.

de Beauvoir, Simone. *The Coming of Age.* Paris: Gallimard, 1970.

Beck, A. T., et al. *Cognitive Therapy for Depression.* New York: Guilford Press, 1979.

Blazer, D. G. "The OARS-Durham Surveys: Description and Application." In *Multi-Dimensional Functional Assessment: The OARS Methodology* (2nd Ed.). Durham, N.C.: Center for the Study of Aging and Human Development, 1978a.

Blazer, D. G. "Techniques for Communicating with your Elderly Patient." *Geriatrics* 33:79, 1978b.

Blazer, D. G. "The Diagnosis of Depression in the Elderly." *Journal of the American Geriatrics Society* 28(2)52, 1980.

Blazer, D. B. "Family Therapy With the Depressed Older Adult." In Blazer, D. G., *Depression in Late Life*. St. Louis: C. V. Mosby, 1982a, pp. 221–235.

Blazer, D. G. *Depression in Late Life*. St. Louis: C. V. Mosby, 1982b.

Blazer, D. G. "Impact of Late Life Depression on the Social Network." *American Journal of Psychiatry* 140:162, 1983.

Blazer D. G., and Williams, C. D. "The Epidemiology of Dysphoria and Depression in an Elderly Population." *American Journal of Psychiatry* 137(4):439, 1980.

Bowman, R. E., and Wolf, R. C. "Plasma 17-hydroxy-corticosteroid Response to ACTH." In Mulatta, M. (ed.), *Dose, Age, Weight and Sex. Proceedings of the Society for Experimental Biology and Medicine*, 130:61, 1969.

Butler, R. "Old Age." In Arieti, S. (ed.), *American Handbook of Psychiatry*, Volume I (2nd Ed.). New York: Basic Books, 1974.

Carroll, B. J., et al. "A Specific Laboratory Test for the Diagnosis of Melancholia: Standardization, Validation and Clinical Utility." *Archives of General Psychiatry* 38:15–22, 1981.

Cassel, J. "The Contribution of the Social Environment to Host Resistance." *American Journal of Epidemiology* 104:107, 1976.

Cheach, K. C., and Beard, O. W. "Psychiatric Findings in the Population of a Geriatric Evaluation Unit: Implications." *Journal of the American Geriatrics Society* 28:153, 1980.

Cole, J. O. "Drug Therapy of Senile Organic Brain Syndromes." *Psychiatric Journal of Ottawa* 5:41, 1980.

Crook, T. "Central Nervous System Stimulants: Appraisal of Use in Geropsychiatric Patients." *Journal of the American Geriatrics Society* 27:476, 1979.

Daniel, R. "A Five Year Study of 693 Psychogeriatric Admissions in Queensland." *Geriatrics* 27(1):132, 1972.

Dohrenwend, B. P., et al. "Measures of Nonspecific Psychological Distress and Other Dimensions of Psychopathology in the General Population." *Archives of General Psychiatry* 37:1229–1236, 1980.

Erikson, E. *Childhood and Society*. New York: Norton, 1950.

Frank, J. D. *Persuasion and Healing*. Baltimore: Johns Hopkins University Press, 1979.

Freud, S. Mourning and Melancholia. 1917. Reprinted in *Collected Papers*, Volume IV. London: Hogarth Press, 1950. pp. 152–172.

Friedel, R. O. "The Diagnosis and Treatment of Autonomous Depression in the Geriatric Patient." *Geriatric Medicine Today* 2:40–51, 1983.

Hopkinson, G. "A Genetic Study of Affective Illness in Patients Over 50." *British Journal of Psychiatry* 110:244, 1964.

Kath, S. "Depletion and Restitution." In Berezin, M. A., and Kath, S. (eds.), *Geriatric Psychiatry*. New York: International Universities Press, 1965.

Kupfer, D. J., et al. "EEG's, Sleep, Depression, and Aging." *Neurobiology of Aging* 3:351, 1982.

Lazarus, L. W., and Weinberg, J. "Treatment in the Ambulatory Care Setting." In Busse, E. W., and Blazer D. G. (eds.), *Handbook of Geriatric Psychiatry*. New York: Van Nostrand Reinhold, 1980, pp. 427–452.

Linn, L. "Clinical Manifestations of Psychiatric Disorders." In Freedman, A. M., Kaplan, H. I., and Sadock, B. J. (eds.), *Comprehensive Textbook of Psychiatry*. Baltimore: Williams and Wilkins, 1975, pp. 783–825.

Loosen, P. T., and Prange, A. J. "Serum Thyrotrophin Response to Thyrotrophin Releasing Hormone in Psychiatric Patients: A Review." *American Journal of Psychiatry* 139:4, 1982.

Loosen, P. T., et al. "Thyroid Stimulating Hormone Response After Thyrotrophin Releasing Hormone in Depressed, Schizophrenic, and Normal Women." *Psychoneuroendocrinology* 2:137, 1977.

Lowenthal, M. F., and Berkman, P. L. *Aging and Mental Disorder in San Francisco: A Social Psychiatric Study.* San Francisco: Jossey-Bass, 1967.

MacMahon, B., and Pugh, T. F. *Epidemiology: Principles and Methods.* Boston: Little, Brown, 1979.

Mendels, J., Stern, S., and Frazer, A. "Biochemistry of Depression." *Diseases of the Nervous System* 37:3, 1976.

Mendlewicz, J. "The Age Factor in Depressive Illness: Some Genetic Consideration." *Journal of Gerontology* 31:300, 1976.

Morris, J. N. *Uses of Epidemiology* (3rd ed.). London: Churchill Livingstone, 1975.

Myers, J. K., et al. "The Prevalence of Psychiatric Disorders in Three Communities 1980–1982." Paper Presented at the Meeting of the American Public Health Association, Montreal, Canada, 1982.

Neugarten, B. L. "Adaptation and the Life Cycle." *Journal of Geriatric Psychology* 4(1):71, 1970.

Nies, A., et al. "Relationship Between Age and Tricyclic Antidepressant Plasma Levels." *American Journal of Psychiatry* 134:790, 1977.

Palmore, E., and Kivett, V. "Changes in Life Satisfaction: A Longitudinal Study of Persons 46–70." *Journal of Gerontology* 32:311, 1970.

Prange, A. J., et al. "Enhancement of Imipramine by Thyroid Stimulating Hormone: Clinical and Theoretical Implications." *American Journal of Psychiatry* 127:191, 1970.

Quitkin, F., Rifkin, A., and Klein, D. F. "Monoamine Oxidase Inhibitors." *Archives of General Psychiatry* 36:749, 1979.

Raskind M., et al. "DST and Cortisol Circadian Rhythm in Primary Degenerative Dementia." *American Journal of Psychiatry* 139:11, 1982.

Ray, W. A., Federspiel, C. F., and Schaffner, W. A. "A Study of Antipsychotic Drug Use in Nursing Homes: Epidemiologic Evidence Suggesting Misuse." *American Journal of Public Health* 70:45, 1980.

Regier, D. A., Goldberg, I. D., and Taube, C. A. "The De Facto U.S. Mental Health Services System." *Archives of General Psychiatry* 35:685, 1978.

Reiser, M. F. "Implications of a Biopsychosocial Model for Research in Psychiatry." *Psychosomatic Medicine* 42 (Supplement):141, 1980.

Samorajski, T., Rosten, C., and Ordy, J. M. "Changes in Behavior, Brain and Neuroendocrine Chemistry with Age and Stress in C 57 BL/6 J Male Mice." *Journal of Gerontology* 26:168, 1971.

Schildkraut, J. J. "Catecholamine Hypothesis of Affective Disorders." *American Journal of Psychiatry* 122:509, 1965.

Seligman, M.E.P. "Depression and Learned Helplessness." In Friedman, J. R., and Katz, M. D. (eds.), *The Psychology of Depression: Contemporary Theory in Research.* Washington, D.C.: Winston, 1974.

Slater, E., and Cowie, V. *The Genetics of Mental Disorders.* London: Oxford University Press, 1971.

Steuer, J. "Psychotherapy for Depressed Elders." In Blazer, D. G., *Depression in Late Life.* St. Louis: C. V. Mosby, 1982, pp. 195–220.

U.S. Department of Health, Education and Welfare. *Vital Statistics of the U.S., 1975.* Washington, D.C, 1978.

Weiner, R. D. "The Role of Electroconvulsive Therapy and the Treatment of Depression in the Elderly." *Journal of the American Geriatrics Society* 30:710, 1982.

Weissman, M. M. and Myers, J. K. "Effective Disorders in a U.S. Urban Community." *Archives of General Psychiatry* 35:1304, 1978.

Wertheimer, J., et al. "Evaluating a Service in Lausanne." In Wing, J. K., and Hafner, H. (eds.), *Routes of Evaluation: The Epidemiological Basis for Planning Psychiatric Services*. London: Oxford University Press, 1973, pp. 257–268.

Wigdor, B. T. "Drives and Motivation with Aging." In Birran, J. E., and Sloane, R. B. (eds.), *Handbook of Mental Health and Aging*. Englewood Cliffs, N.J.: Prentice-Hall, 1980, pp. 245–261.

Aging and Age-Dependent Disease:
Cognition and Dementia

Robert Katzman*

A major characteristic of aging is an increase in heterogeneity of the population. Some individuals remain relatively intact; others succumb to one or another age-related disease. This is well illustrated when changes in cognition are considered. At age 80, about half of the population is still cognitively "normal." Some 80- and even 90-year-olds may be extraordinarily productive; consider such examples as Eubie Blake, Pablo Casals, Picasso, Conrad Adenauer, Rebecca West, and Grandma Moses, individuals who remained productive late in life. At the same time a significant proportion of individuals in their 80s and 90s develop serious diseases of the brain, particularly Alzheimer's disease and cerebrovascular disease, which can lead to progressive loss of cognitive processes to the point where individuals become completely dependent, lose their identity as individuals, and become true "geriatric tragedies" (Figure 1). It is the purpose of this paper to delineate the differences between the normal aging processes that may affect cognition and diseases that are age-dependent and can devastate the brain and lead to total incapacity.

*Professor and Chairman, Department of Neurology, Albert Einstein College of Medicine, Montefiore Medical Center, New York, New York.

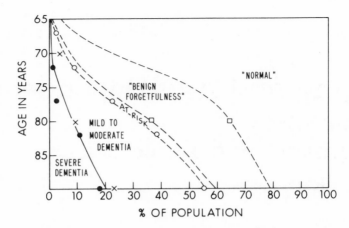

FIGURE 1   The changing pattern of cognitive abilities and dementia as a
function of age: a hypothetical projection. The data points shown are based
upon: x, the prevalence of "severe" dementia at different ages in Syracuse,
New York,[35] ●, prevalence of "severe" and ○, "mild" dementia on the Island
of Samso, Denmark,[36] and □, pattern of mental status changes in an 80-
year-old cohort, Bronx Aging Study. (See text for definition of terms.)

NORMAL AGING AND COGNITION

Cognitive changes do, of course, occur with aging, even among
those free of serious brain disease. As most individuals age, and
particularly as they reach their 70s or 80s, they notice an increase
in mild forgetfulness, a difficulty in remembering proper names.
Tasks requiring new learning may be more difficult and take
more time, but can often be mastered. All aspects of life become
somewhat slower. It becomes easier to focus on one task rather
than trying to manipulate a variety of different tasks simultaneously. All of the changes commonly observed occur as part of
the normal aging of the brain. One of the consequences of normal
aging is a shrinkage of the brain and a loss of nerve cells. Autopsy
series show that the weight of the brain in individuals past age
70 is about 10 percent less than the weight of the brain of individuals age 30.[1] There has been some criticism of these data
on the grounds that changes in nutrition and health that occurred
at the turn of the century may have actually increased the size
of the brain, so that in comparing the brains of individuals born,
for example, in 1890 and 1950, one must take into account generational or cohort differences. Indeed Corsellis,[2] checking brain

weights of individuals who died at age 30 but were born between 1870 and 1940, demonstrated an approximately 5 percent increase in brain weight. However, even when this is taken into account there is certainly a shrinkage of the brain on the basis of both numerical averages and the changes in the ratio of brain volume to total intracranial skull volume that occurs during aging.[3,4] This is seen dramatically on the computed tomography (CT) scan, which shows some degree of brain atrophy in apparently normal individuals as a function of age.[5,6] There is considerable variation in brain weights of elderly subjects (70 to 89 years old) known to be cognitively intact during life, their brain weights ranging from 930 to 1,350 g.[7]

In addition to these volume changes, cell counts show a loss of 10 to 50 percent of nerve cells in various areas of the brain, although there are a number of groups of nerve cells in the brain stem which are spared from cell loss, particularly those groups serving a motor function for eye movements.[8] Nerve cells in the cerebral cortex are lost to a variable degree, the greatest loss occurring in the temporal gyrus.[9] In the cerebral cortex the major loss is that of the large cells which project to other regions of the brain; small interneurons seem to survive quite well.

The changes that occur in normal aging must be examined in the context of the overall development of the brain. As the brain is initially formed during late embryogenesis through the postnatal period, the process of cell division leads to formation of new nerve cells which migrate to appropriate regions of the brain. The total nerve cells thus formed are often twice the number needed for functioning of the brain. Some nerve cells fail to make suitable connections; others may be superfluous for other reasons. In any event, during the period when the total brain mass is growing, as processes are being elaborated, the actual number of nerve cells decreases rather significantly. A good example are the number of cells in the substantia nigra, the region of the brain affected by Parkinson's disease. The substantia nigra ("black substance") is composed of a group of pigmented nerve cells deep in the midbrain; these nerve cells, which contain dopamine as a neurotransmitter, send many processes to form connections within the basal ganglia. The substantia nigra plays a major role in ordinary motor activity, and disease of the substantia nigra leads to the changes in gait, posture, and fine movements of parkinsonism. Investigators have counted the number of cells within the substantia nigra in human brain systems at different ages.[10] There is a loss of nerve cells between the ages of 30 and 80, but there is an even greater loss before this period as part of the natural development and maturation of the brain. Thus, changes that occur in normal aging must be considered in the context of a dynamic developmental process beginning early in life. The problem, of course, is that in adult life nerve cells lose the capacity to divide, so that if there is excessive loss of nerve cells there is no way of replacing them. Hence it is conceivable that the very genetic programs that lead to elimination of unneeded nerve cells may continue leading to the loss of nerve cells essential for full performance.

The functional effect of this loss of nerve cells in normal aging is surprisingly small. Longitudinal studies have demonstrated that most aspects of the functions that we consider to represent intelligence remain intact throughout life and indeed may show improvement during maturation.[7] For example, Owens[11] identified a group of men who, at about the age of 19 and in the year 1919, had taken the army alpha test, an examination roughly corresponding to intelligence tests now in more common use. Owens retested these former University of Iowa freshmen in 1950 and again in 1961 and found that performance in the army alpha test improved between the ages of 19 and 50 was quite stable between the ages of 50 and 61. Performance actually showed most improvement on tests measuring vocabulary, information, and comprehension. A study conducted at the National Institute of Mental Health (NIMH) in the mid-1950s identified a group of volunteers, primarily professionals, who were then followed for a period of 11 years.[12] The average age of the volunteers when the study began was about 70, and individuals were followed to an average age of 81. Again, there was relative stability in test findings with some apparent improvement in the verbal intelligence scales, including vocabulary and information. However, a number of timed tests did show some decrement, a finding commented on below. The NIMH study has been criticized because the group of volunteers were said to be "super normals" and not representative of normal aging. However, quite similar longitudinal studies in Hamburg[13] and Bonn,[14] Germany, involving primarily lower middle class subjects showed essentially the same findings. Schiae and co-workers followed members of a health maintenance organization in Puget Sound, Washington, and found again that primary abilities involving verbal functions remained unchanged for a 14-year follow-up period even though individuals initially entering this study were in their 60s.[15,16]

It must be noted that these findings from longitudinal studies are in conflict with evidence from cross sectional studies. The largest cross-sectional study of intelligence as a function of age, involving a true population sample, was the 1955 standardization of the Wechsler Adult Intelligence Scale.[17] A rather dramatic difference in mean test scores even in such areas as vocabulary and information was found between subjects in their 20s and subjects over the age of 55. However, these groups were not comparable in education. Reflecting as they did the average experience of their own generation, individuals who at the time of this study were 55 had been born in 1900 and two-thirds had had only an eighth grade education, whereas among 20-year-olds in the same study, born in 1935, 82 percent had entered and most had finished high school.[18] Education clearly plays a major role in performance on intelligence tests and most of the differences between ages in test performance may represent differences in educational experience. Recognizing the impact of education and other socioeconomic factors on intelligence testing, psychologists who use cross-sectional data in order to answer questions in a brief period of time now attempt to equate younger and older groups in terms of educational background. Such equating can never be precise but is the best that can be done.

Although intelligence tests show that vocabulary, information, comprehension, and aspects of intelligence that have been called "crystallized" intelligence[19] do not change appreciably over adult life, other psychological functions certainly do. Timed tests, those that measure the speed of processing by the brain, clearly show a decrement, particularly past the age of 60. Birren and co-workers have suggested that this is a generalized aging process in the brain affecting many behaviors.[20]

The fact that one slows down during maturation and aging is accepted in sports. Thus the records for the fastest 100-yard dash and the fastest marathon are held by athletes in their early 20s, although some record milers have been somewhat older.[21] The 1980 New York marathon was won by a 22-year-old in less than 2 hours and 10 minutes; a 76-year-old participant required 3 hours and 40 minutes to complete the marathon. Nevertheless an extraordinary degree of overlap occurs between younger and older individuals. The time for the 76-year-old who was able to complete the marathon in under 4 hours is still much faster than the time of many 20-year-olds, and of course the majority of the population at any age could not complete the 26-mile distance in a reasonable time. It has been found that 70-year-olds who engage actively in running or racquet sports have reaction times that are faster than those of 20-year-olds who lead sedentary lives. As a group, however, 70-year-olds are significantly slower than 20-year-olds.

The slowing that occurs with aging is primarily due to a slowing of central processing by the brain.[22] The age decrement in choice reaction time is much greater than that of simple reaction time; the difference is due to lengthening in central processing rather than to perceptual or motor abilities. This slowing on a central basis that occurs with aging can also be demonstrated by measures of electrophysiological events. Electrophysiological signals determined by averaging cortical brain waves can be used to identify the arrival of a perceptual signal into the primary sensory area of the brain, and subsequent waves can be used to identify various signal elements, central processing of such signals, and initiation of a motor response. It is clear that the late components of these sensory evoked responses are markedly delayed in older subjects compared to reasonably matched younger subjects. The anatomic basis for this slowing is not understood, but might reflect loss of the synapses that occurs as part of normal aging.

A second process significantly affected in normal aging is episodic short-term memory.[23] When older and younger subjects are asked to remember a list of digits, nonsense syllables, or unrelated words, the ability to do so markedly decreases with age.[24] In part, this loss can be reversed if the older subjects are taught strategies for memorizing, but the reversal is never complete.[25] On the other hand, when materials with true semantic value are presented—for example, ideas—older subjects will learn the ideas as well as younger subjects do.[26] Thus, semantic learning appears to be minimally affected, whereas episodic short-term memory is seriously affected.

The mechanisms underlying the deficit in episodic short-term memory are not fully understood. Problems with both learning and retrieval appear to be involved. One contributing factor may also be the loss of processing speed; this can be demonstrated using the Sternberg paradigm, in which the speed of response in selecting a word previously assigned from a group of words is measured.[27] As the initial group of words to be learned is increased in number, all subjects take a longer and longer period to choose the correct word. The increase in time, however, is exaggerated in older subjects, again evidence of loss of processing speed.[28] However, it is probable that factors other than speed of processing are involved in age decrements and memory.

Older individuals often have difficulty with complex materials.[29] It is more difficult for older subjects to perform several tasks simultaneously. This has been described variously as a problem in "channel capacity," in "attention," or in "cognitive effort." Psychological methods for studying these changes are currently being developed and may provide interesting data on normal aging processes that will add to our understanding of age changes.[30]

While intelligence, in terms of vocabulary, information, and comprehension, is stable over most of adult life, there is some question as to whether decrements in these areas occur in individuals past 75. Here the data are not consistent. The evidence from the NIMH study suggests that there is no decrement for most individuals. Data from the Duke Longitudinal study[31] and the Kalman twin study[32] suggest that indeed there is some loss, even in these areas of "crystallized intelligence," past the age of 75. An important methodologic problem is that in subjects past the age of 75 a significant percentage may be developing one or another of the diseases that devastate cognition. If such a change occurring in a percentage of a cohort is unrecognized, then the "average" performance will show decline. To resolve this question it would be necessary to follow individuals beyond the re-test in order to identify those who are at an early stage in the process of developing dementia.

DEMENTIA AND DISEASES THAT PRODUCE DEMENTIA

The term "dementia," although used widely in common parlance, has a specific medical meaning. Dementia is defined in the third edition of the *Diagnostic and Statistical Manual* (DSM III) of the American Psychiatric Association[33] as follows: "A loss of intellectual abilities of sufficient severity to interfere with social or occupational functioning; memory impairment; at least one of the following—impairment of abstract thinking . . . inability to find similarities and differences between related words, difficulty in defining words and concepts, and other similar tasks, impaired judgment, other disturbances of higher cortical function, such as aphasia . . . apraxia . . . constructional difficulty . . . personality change; a state of consciousness not clouded."

There is an interesting background to this definition. The symptom complex it describes had been called dementia for many decades by physicians. However, in 1952 the American Psychiatric Association, in the first edition of its diagnostic and statistical manual, coined a new phrase, "chronic organic brain syndrome," to replace the term dementia. The invention of this phrase created a split in American medicine between neurologists and other physicians who continued to use the term dementia and their psychiatric brethren. The term "chronic organic brain syndrome" was dropped from psychiatric jargon in 1980 with the publication of DSM III.

Community surveys seeking to identify the problems of dementia normally use a variation of this definition, together with the mental status test, to determine the actual extent of memory and other cognitive deficits. Such surveys have shown that between 4 and 5 percent of individuals over the age of 65 are demented to the degree that they can no longer live independently and require care in either a nursing home or similar institution, or require relatively full-time care by their families.[34] This group is said to have "severe dementia." Individuals with mild to moderate impairment who are still able to function in the community constitute roughly 10 percent of individuals over the age of 65. However, prevalence is very much age-related so that the percent of individuals with severe dementia in the population over 85 will be in the range of 15 to 20 percent[35,36] (see Figure 1). These prevalence figures have been obtained in studies involving community surveys, that is, cross-sectional population surveys based either on interviews to ascertain the health of individuals or, in the case of studies from Scandinavia, on review of relatively complete medical files on such individuals.

Incidence figures for dementia have not been available until recently, but there are now some data from two longitudinal studies: the Baltimore Longitudinal Study[37] and the study in Lundby, Sweden, carried out by Hagnell et al.[38] They also indi-

cate a sharp rise in incidence with age, reaching a figure of between 3 and 4 percent per year in individuals in their 80s. Inter-
estingly, the Hagnell data show a fall-off in individuals in their
90s, the yearly incidence falling below 2 percent (Figure 2).

We are currently following a group of 400 80-year-old, nonde-
mented volunteers with yearly health evaluations that include
tests of mental status and neurological and neuropsychological
functioning—the Bronx Aging Study. In our first follow-up we
have found that 6 percent show a major change in cognitive
ability, with 4 percent becoming demented during this 1-year
period, in accord with the incidence reported in the Lundby study.

However, a surprisingly large number of "normal" 80-year-
olds in our study show evidence of difficulty with simple memory
tasks such as recall of a name and address several minutes after
learning them, and recall of two lists of 10 or 12 objects even
when the objects have been touched, visualized, and named. Kral
in 1962[39] noted this large subgroup and followed it for several
years; in most, neither premature death nor a true dementia

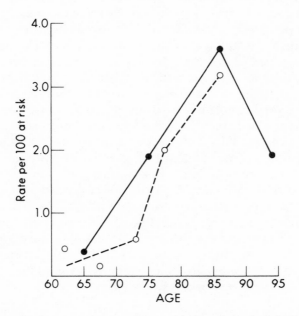

FIGURE 2   Incidence of development of dementia per 100 individuals at
risk per year. ●, Data of Hagnell for women in Lundby study.[38] ○, Data of
Sluss et al.[37] for men in Baltimore Longitudinal Study.

developed. In the Bronx Aging Study 40 percent of the 80-year-old volunteers resembled 60-year-olds in their performance on a 32-item mental status test,* making no or only one error. Fifty percent made two to five errors, primarily on the memory phase. These individuals, forgetful on testing, did seem to have a benign course, since only 1.5 percent developed dementia the next year, comparable to those making no to one error. However, individuals making six to eight errors were at high risk for (or already in the early stages of) dementia, 15 percent becoming frankly demented within a year. Thus, it now becomes possible to identify those 80-year-olds at high risk for dementia while they are still functioning independently in the community.

Dementia is a symptom complex and may be caused by a variety of diseases. Haase, in Wells's monograph on dementia, has listed over 50 diseases that may produce dementia.[41] In both pathologic and clinical series[42–45] it has been found that Alzheimer's disease is responsible for well over 50 percent of all cases of dementia. Vascular diseases produce dementia when there have been multiple strokes; when more than 50 to 100 g of brain tissue in the cerebral hemisphere have been destroyed or infarcted because of vascular occlusions, dementia usually ensues.[46] Since the amount of brain tissue infarcted is important and the degree of arteriosclerosis of cerebral blood vessels per se is not correlated with dementia, the term "cerebral arteriosclerosis" has been dropped and dementia of vascular origin is termed "multi-infarct dementia." Multi-infarct dementia had been found to account for 20 percent of cases of dementia in series from the 1960s and early 1970s, but its prevalence is decreasing with the dramatic fall in the incidence of strokes in the last 15 years. Another 10 percent of older individuals with dementia have a mixture of Alzheimer's and multi-infarct dementia disease.

In the remaining 20 to 25 percent of individuals with dementia, a wide variety of disorders must be considered in the differential diagnosis. Some of these less common disorders are quite treatable, for example, thyroid deficiency, thiamine (vitamin B_1) deficiency, and vitamin B_{12} deficiency. Thus, a complete blood work-up and metabolic screen are necessary. Moreover, in pathologic series studied before the advent of the CT scan, between 4 and

---

*The test used was a modification of the information–concentration–orientation test previously validated by Blessed et al.[40] by clinical pathological correlation.

5 percent of all patients presenting with dementia turned out to have undiagnosed brain tumors.[44] Another 1 percent of patients with dementia were found to have hydrocephalus, a condition that can be treated by placing a shunt into the enlarged cerebral ventricles in order to divert excess spinal fluid away from the intracranial compartment. Also, some patients with dementia have undiagnosed collections of blood called subdural hematomas, another surgically treatable disorder. Brain tumors, hydrocephalus, and subdural hematomas are all easily identified on a CT scan and for that reason the CT scan becomes a necessary part of the work-up of a patient with dementia. Alzheimer patients as a group have a greater degree of brain atrophy than do age-matched controls. Although the CT scan may be used to estimate the degree of atrophy, because there is so much variation in the degree of atrophy in normal individuals during aging and among those with Alzheimer's disease, this use of the CT scan is not a reliable diagnostic aid.

The overall work-up required for a differential diagnosis of dementia is shown in Table 1. Costing between $800 and $1,200, it is a relatively expensive work-up. However, when one considers that the majority of individuals in nursing homes are there be-

TABLE 1   Work-up for Differential Diagnosis of Dementia

Examination	Cost	
	Low	High
By the examiner: history, mental status, physical condition, and neurological condition	$125	$200
Special tests		
CT scan	200	
High resolution		350
Chest x-ray study	25	45
Electrocardiogram	35	45
Electroencephalogram		
Routine	70	
Quantitative		150
Blood studies		
Complete blood cell count; metabolic screen thyroid profile; B_{12} level; VDRL[a]	90	120
Psychometric evaluation	250	350
Total	$795	$1,260

[a]Test for syphilis.

cause they have developed dementia and cannot be cared for in society, the cost benefit of identifying even a few percent of individuals with treatable dementias who might be spared nursing home care is great. Thus, the current annual cost of nursing home care is about 30 billion dollars; if 60 percent of this is ascribed to the presence of dementia, that cost is 18 billion dollars per year. Reducing nursing home occupancy by 2 percent would amount to 360 million dollars. There are about 350,000 new patients with dementia each year, so that the cost of their work-up would in fact be paid for if there were about a 2 percent reduction in nursing home placement. And this does not take into account the economic savings to families who care for over half of all end-stage dementia patients. Thus, on a purely economic basis, a full work-up is justified even without taking into account the significant social benefit to be derived by identifying reversible cases of dementia.

ALZHEIMER'S DISEASE

From a public health point of view, there is no doubt that Alzheimer's disease has already become a major health problem, accounting for at least 55 percent of cases of senile dementia. With over 600,000 individuals severely afflicted in the United States and requiring either nursing home care or its equivalent in the community, and with another estimated million individuals in earlier phases of the disorder, the importance of the disease becomes apparent. Lewis Thomas[47] describes it as "quite epidemic." With the incidence of Alzheimer's disease about 3 percent per year in individuals in their mid-80s and with the rapid increase in the number of individuals at risk that is occurring because of our improved ability to prevent and treat cardiovascular disease and stroke (there has been a 20 percent decrease in mortality in the 85+ population during the past decade[48]), there is every expectation that Alzheimer's disease will become even more important as a health problem.

Underlying such statements is the consensus that has developed that the condition recognized for many years as a "presenile dementia" is identical to the disease that produces the majority of cases of senile dementia.[49] In accord with this assumption is the similarity in basic clinical presentation of Alzheimer's disease at any age. The disease usually begins insidiously with the family somewhat uncertain as to when symptoms first appeared. Usually memory is involved first, but sometimes the affected individual has difficulty in finding words, becomes lost, and loses things. Symptoms continue to progress with more and more areas of cognition becoming involved. The ability to perform complex tasks such as balancing a checkbook or handling fiscal affairs is among the first to fail, but as progression continues, simple tasks (preparing a meal, shopping, playing cards, remembering appointments) are lost; sometimes the patient may become depressed or agitated, speech becomes sparse, dressing and eating become difficult to carry out, and incontinence begins. (Younger patients more often may show difficulty with language and spatial tasks, and older patients with memory, but the generalization does not hold up well.) The patient eventually becomes fully dependent and unreactive. This course of events may take from 1 to 20 years. Life expectancy is reduced by half from the time of onset of the disease.

Alois Alzheimer, a psychiatrist, neurologist, and neuropathologist at the turn of the century, first applied a newly discovered silver stain to microscopic sections of the brain of a patient with a progressive fatal dementia that had begun at age 51.[50] Alzheimer discovered the presence of grossly abnormal nerve cells filled with tangles of fibrillary material. These abnormal cells are called neurofibrillary tangles; silver-staining foci within the brain tissue are termed neuritic plaques. These neuropathologic features are present in the brains of patients who develop the disease in their 50s and 60s and also in patients who die of the disease during the senium.[51]

In 1964, Terry[52] identified the electronmicroscopic characteristics of the neurofibrillary tangle and neuritic plaque and found them to be identical in the brains of younger and older individuals.[53] The neurofibrillary tangle is composed not of a small number of abnormal fibrils as it appears to be under the light microscope, but instead contains tens of thousands of abnormal filaments with two filaments 100 Å in diameter wound around each other to form a paired helical filament.[54] This filament is unique for homo sapiens and there is no equivalent in experimental animals, not even in very old primates. The neuritic plaque was shown by Terry to be composed of degenerating nerve terminals, in many instances still forming synapses. In addition there is an increase in supporting cells, including glial and microglial cells, in the neuritic plaque. The degenerating terminals surround a protein core that has the characteristic of amyloid, a beta-pleated fibrillar protein present in a number of chronic diseases elsewhere in the body but probably of unique origin in the brain of the Alzheimer patient.

Neurofibrillary tangles and neuritic plaques may be present in the brains of normal individuals who die. In Alzheimer's disease the neurofibrillary tangles and neuritic plaques are found abundantly in the cerebral cortex and in the hippocampus and amygdala, whereas during normal aging a few tangles and plaques are found in the hippocampus and an occasional plaque in the cerebal cortex. It remained, however, for a prospective study carried out by Blessed, Tomlinson, and Roth in Newcastle, England, to demonstrate that the number of plaques in the cerebral cortex and the presence of neurofibrillary tangles in the cortex correlated very well with the presence of dementia during life.[40,42] These authors found a correlation ($r = .7$) between dementia score determined during life and the number of neuritic plaques counted in several areas of the cerebral cortex. This was indeed extraordinary since the sampling error is potentially very great, considering the minute size of the microscopic sections examined as compared to the entire volume of the cerebral cortex. This finding has been confirmed in other studies.[55] Thus, the degree of intellectual deterioration in Alzheimer's disease is correlated with the extent of the pathologic change in the brain.

In 1976, three laboratories independently discovered the existence of a relatively specific biochemical change in the brains of patients with Alzheimer's disease.[56–58] Choline acetyltransferase is an enzyme that converts choline plus acetate into acetylcholine, a chemical used by some nerve cells to signal other nerve cells, that is, a neurotransmitter. Acetylcholine is only one of perhaps 30 chemicals that may have the role of neurotransmitter in the brain. However, in Alzheimer's disease there is a marked reduction, sometimes of the order of 90 percent, in the amount of this enzyme in the cerebral cortex and hippocampus, the areas of the brain affected pathologically. Other parts of the brain that contain acetylcholine such as the basal ganglia have little or no reduction in the choline acetyltransferase. This finding became even more intriguing when it was discovered that the receptor for acetylcholine, on the postsynaptic cell where acetylcholine acts, is spared.[58,59]

How specific, how important clinically is the reduction in choline acetyltransferase? When the cholinergic antagonist that acts by blocking the muscarinic receptor in the brain, scopolamine, is given to normal volunteers, a state of confusion and amnesia develops that resembles in many respects a moderately demented Alzheimer patient.[60,61] Scopolamine, in fact, was used for many years to produce the state of "twilight sleep" in women during delivery, the mother then forgetting her pain. Also, Perry et al.[62] compared the degree of dementia in Alzheimer patients with postmortem measurement of choline acetyltransferase and found an excellent correlation.

Of 14 additional transmitters that have now been studied, only one, somatostatin, a neuropeptide present in the cerebral cortex, has been found to be reduced in a consistent fashion.[63] In some cases noradrenalin is reduced in Alzheimer's disease.[64] Vasoactive intestinal peptide and cholecystokinin, two of the major neuropeptide transmitters in the cerebral cortex, are quite normal in the Alzheimer brain.[65] The major inhibitory system, the gamma-aminobutyric acid neurons, is spared in the Alzheimer brain.[66]

It is interesting to note that discovery of the clinical importance of the cholinergic system in Alzheimer's disease has led to basic research on the anatomy of the system, and it has been found that over 70 percent of the choline acetyltransferase in the cerebral cortex is present in nerve endings that project into the cerebral cortex from a nucleus deep in the basal forebrain, the basal nucleus of Meynert.[66] It has now been reported that the number of nerve cells in the basal nucleus of Meynert is reduced by as much as 80 percent in Alzheimer cases.[67] Much of the choline acetyltransferase in the other region of the brain most affected, the hippocampus, is present in the nerve endings arising from nerve processes projecting from the septal nucleus, the region of the brain contiguous to the basal nucleus of Meynert. Thus, a system of deep forebrain cholinergic nerve cells projecting to the cerebral cortex and hippocampus provides one key to Alzheimer's disease.

But this cannot be the only key. The large nerve cells in the hippocampus and cerebral cortex that develop into neurofibrillary tangles are not cholinergic. Terry et al.[68] have shown that in the frontal, temporal, and parietal cerebral cortex in Alzheimer brains, there is a loss of very large ($90\text{-}\mu m^2$ in cross-sectional area) nerve cells, by as much as 50 percent, compared to the same brain regions of age-matched normals. Part of this loss could well be due to the loss of somatostatin cells, but somatostatin would not account for all the large cells. We do not know which other neurotransmitter-specific cells are vulnerable to the Alzheimer process; such information would be valuable, since it might point the way to a reasonable working hypothesis as to what causes the death of the neurotransmitter-specific cells. Is it a genetically programmed event? An exogenous toxin such as aluminum? A slow virus? An endogenous toxin such as an excitatory neurotransmitter? An antibody to a subclass of cerebral cortical neurons? Loss of a factor (trophic factor) needed to sustain the life of the cell?

With these pathological and biochemical findings Alzheimer's disease takes on the characteristics of other medical diseases. For the greater part of this century most individuals who developed senile dementia were said to have cerebral arteriosclerosis. The degree of arteriosclerosis of the great vessels that act as conduits of blood to the brain were shown by Corsellis[69] to be unrelated to the degree of dementia. But there has always been a nagging feeling by various investigators that perhaps a deficiency in oxygen or blood supply might underlie the development of even the Alzheimer changes. There is certainly no clinical basis for such a belief in younger patients with Alzheimer's disease; most are in quite excellent health, and many are able to continue to engage in athletics well into the course of their dementing illness (motor areas are spared by the Alzheimer process). However, it was not until the development of positron emission tomography that it became possible to demonstrate that there is no abnormality in the utilization of oxygen in the Alzheimer brain,[70] although the total demand for oxygen is reduced as the brain functions less well and does not have to metabolize oxygen and sugar to the extent that it did when it was at full activity.

The discovery of a relatively specific biochemical deficit in Alzheimer's disease, although probably but one of several yet to be discovered, has led a number of investigators to seek ways of treating this deficit by administering precursors such as choline or lecithin, or by administering drugs such as physostigmine that block the breakdown of the acetylcholine still produced in the brain. Precursor therapy has been found to be unavailing,[71] but physostigmine does improve memory to some extent.[72,73] Unfortunately it does not improve other behavioral changes in the

Alzheimer patient, nor does it affect the course of the disease. However, the fact that there is some effect on memory is encouraging and ought to lead to the development of much more potent drugs, perhaps including cholinergic agonists that can act directly on the brain of the Alzheimer patient. More important if we are to prevent Alzheimer's disease, however, is to discover its cause. We do not understand the risk factors for this disorder. The only risk factor that has been relatively well defined is genetic predisposition. There is a small subset of families in whom the disease appears to be inherited in a dominant pattern.[74] If one has a first degree relative—that is a father, mother, brother, or sister—with Alzheimer's disease, one's chances of developing this disorder are increased three- to fourfold at a given age. This was found in both a Swedish and a Minnesota study.[75,76] However, the majority of cases are sporadic, that is, the disease occurs in individuals who do not have a family history of it.

Concordance in identical twins is only about 50 percent.[77] Cook and co-workers reported two identical twins who developed Alzheimer's disease confirmed at autopsy.[78] One twin developed the disease in her late 60s, while the second twin had no symptoms before age 82. The 13 to 15 year difference between these two twins in the age at which symptoms began has led these authors to question the lack of concordance in Alzheimer twins, and to speculate that perhaps, in some sets of twins, the second twin had not been followed long enough for the investigator to be sure that Alzheimer's disease would not develop. However, one can interpret this finding otherwise; that is, that there must be some risk factors other than genetic that delayed the onset of the disease in one twin by 15 years. Indeed, if one knew what these factors were and could delay the onset of the disease by a period of 15 years, Alzheimer's disease would disappear as a public health problem given the current maximum life span. Thus, identification of risk factors other than a genetic one would seem to be an important goal.

There is an intriguing but as yet not well understood relationship between Down's syndrome (mongolism, or trisomy 21) and Alzheimer's disease. Individuals with Down's syndrome who live to the age of 40 almost invariably develop Alzheimer-like changes in the brain, often in association with a behavioral disturbance that must represent the equivalent of a dementia in an individual who is already intellectually impaired.[79,80] The brains of Down's syndrome patients show not only the presence of neurofibrillary tangles and neuritic plaques, but also the loss of choline acetyltransferase as in the Alzheimer counterpart.[81] There is no evidence of an abnormality in chromosome 21 in Alzheimer patients; yet it would appear that a genetic change because of the extra chromosome is a sufficient although not a necessary cause of the Alzheimer process. An intriguing facet of this problem is that a small increase has been noted in the number of individuals with Down's syndrome in families with Alzheimer probands, although this is not a consistent finding.[82]

To date, investigations of viruses, heavy metals, and other environmental risk factors have been inconclusive. Accumulation of aluminum in the brains of Alzheimer patients has been reported in studies from Canada[83] and Vermont,[84] but not from Kentucky,[85] where the water supply has a very low aluminum content, suggesting that aluminum deposition may have been a secondary finding. Immunologic changes sometimes occur in Alzheimer patients, but these may be secondary rather than primary.

Epidemiological studies looking for other types of risk factors are currently underway, but preliminary data have not been encouraging in believing that a cause will be found using the typical case–control study methodology. It is striking that we know little about the epidemiology of this disease beyond Western Europe, the United States, and Japan. It might be very important to know whether there are populations essentially free of Alzheimer's disease in other parts of the world. Unfortunately this has not been studied, probably because problems of aging have not been important in third world countries in the past, and although such problems are beginning to be seen as important in newly developed countries as their populations age, cooperation in such studies has apparently become more and more difficult. This is an area where new mechanisms for collaborative work must be developed.

There are a number of issues concerning Alzheimer's disease that need to be addressed:

1. The major need is for prevention of the disorder. In order to accomplish this we must learn its cause, a goal that will require extensive research activity. At present, research expenditures on Alzheimer's disease by the federal government are about $22 million. The cost of the disorder in health care expenditures alone

has been estimated at $26 billion; thus, research is one-tenth of 1 percent of the cost of our present, quite inadequate care. Clearly, research support must be increased.

2. Another major need is to find a specific clinical diagnostic procedure or marker to identify Alzheimer patients more accurately during life.

3. We must determine whether a diagnostic work-up should be required before admission to a nursing home, to assure that patients with primary depression or treatable diseases presenting as dementia will be identified and treated.

4. Our society must develop better models of care for the Alzheimer patient, since we do not yet have a way of preventing or treating the disorder. Models that do not require full-time nursing home care—for example, respite services for families and day care centers—are being developed and must be encouraged.

5. A mechanism for attacking several of these problems simultaneously is needed. One might be to establish centers of excellence having clinical demonstration units together with a staff of basic scientists working on the problem.

6. Mechanisms for international cooperation in studies seeking risk factors must be developed.

7. The extraordinary burdens of the families of Alzheimer patients must be addressed. There is an economic burden because Medicare does not pay for the care of patients with chronic diseases such as Alzheimer's disease (most nursing home patients are on Medicaid). There is also a tremendous social burden on the family, particularly if a family member acts as care-giver. At the least, our medical care system should be rationalized so that Medicare instead of Medicaid pays for the costs of Alzheimer's disease. At present, depending upon the jurisdiction in which the patient lives, a couple must either split its resources or "spend down" half of its resources so that the sick individual will be entitled to Medicaid, otherwise both may become paupers. It is a double tragedy.

8. On the other hand, since successful prevention of Alzheimer's disease might materially increase life expectancy, planning must take place to assure that this will not be an economic burden by itself.

9. The tacit asumption in our society that everyone will eventually become "senile" must be put aside. The expected norm should be that of a vigorous, intellectually active aging process.

Productive years could be increased well past current arbitrary retirement ages for many.

REFERENCES

1. Dekaban, A. S., and Sadowsky, D. Changes in brain weights during the span of human life: Relation of brain weight to body heights and body weights. *Ann Neurol* 4:345-365, 1978.

2. Corsellis, J. A. N. Some observations on the purkinje cell population and on brain volume in human aging. In Terry, R. D., and Gershon, S. (eds.), Aging, Vol. 7: *Neurobiology of Aging*. New York: Raven Press, 1978, p. 397.

3. Davis, P.J.M., and Wright, E. A.: A new method for measuring cranial cavity volume and its application to the assessment of cerebral atrophy at autopsy. *Neuropathol Appl Neurobiol*; *3*:341-358, 1977.

4. Terry, R. D., Peck, A., De Teresa, R., Schechter, R., and Horoupian, D. S. Some morphometric aspects of the brain in senile dementia of the Alzheimer type. *Ann Neurol 10*:184, 1981.

5. Glydensted, C. Measurements of the normal ventricular system and hemispheric sulci of 100 adults with computed tomography. *Neuroradiology 14*:183, 1977.

6. Jacoby, R. J., Levy, R., and Dawson, J. M. Computed tomography in the elderly: I. The normal population. *Br J Psychiatry 136*:249, 1980.

7. Katzman, R., and Terry, R. Normal aging of the nervous system. In Katzman, R., and Terry, R. (eds.), *Neurology of Aging*. Philadelphia: F. A. Davis, 1983, pp. 15-49.

8. Konigsmark, B. W., and Murphy, E. A. Volume of ventral cochlear nucleus in man: Its relationship to neuronal population and age. *J Neuropathol Exp Neurol 31*:304, 1972.

9. Brody, Harold: Organization of the cerebral cortex. III. A study of aging in the human cerebral cortex. *J Comp Neurol 102*:511-556, 1955.

10. McGeer, E. G. Aging and neurotransmitter metabolism in the human brain. In Katzman, R., Terry, R. D., and Bick, K. L. (eds.), Aging, Vol. 7: *Alzheimer's Disease: Senile Dementia and Related Disorders*. New York: Raven Press, 1978, p. 427.

11. Owens, W. A. Age and mental abilities: A second adult follow-up. *J Educ Psychol 57*:311, 1966.

12. Granick, S. Psychological test functioning. In Granick, S., and Patterson, R. D. (eds.), *Human Aging II*. Rockville, Md.: U.S. Department of Health, Education and Welfare, DHEW Publication No. (HSM) 71-9037, 1971.

13. Riegel, K. F., Riegel, R. M., and Meyer, G. Socio-psychological factors of aging: A cohort-sequential analysis. *Hum Dev 10*:27, 1967.

14. Thomae, H. *Patterns of Aging*. New York: S. Karger, 1976, p. 1.

15. Schaie, K. W., and Labouvie-Vief, G. Generational versus ontogenetic components of change in adult cognitive behavior: A fourteen-year cross-sequential study. *Dev Psychol*; *10*:305-320, 1974.

16. Schaie, K. W., Labouvie, G. V., and Buech, B. U. Generational and cohort-specific differences in adult cognitive functioning: A fourteen-year study of independent samples. *Dev Psychol 9*:151-166, 1973.

17. Wechsler, D. (ed.). *The Measurement and Appraisal of Adult Intelligence*. 4th Ed. Baltimore: Williams & Wilkins, 1958, p. 297.

18. Wechsler, D. (ed.). *Manual for the Wechsler Adult Intelligence Scale*. New York: The Psychological Corporation, 1955, p. 75.

19. Cattell, R. B. *Abilities: Their Structure, Growth, and Action.* Boston: Houghton Mifflin, 1971.

20. Birren, J. E., Woods, A. M., and Williams, M. V. Speed of behavior as an indicator of age changes and the integrity of the nervous sytem. In Hoffmeister, F., and Muller, C. (eds.), *Brain Function in Old Age.* Berlin: Springer-Verlag, 1979, pp. 10-44.

21. Clark, T. The Masters Movement: Age conquers some, but it doesn't conquer all. *Runner's World,* July, pp. 80-95, 1979.

22. Birren, J. E. Age changes in speed of behavior: Its central nature and physiological correlates. In Welford, A. T., and Birren, J. E. (eds.), *Behavior, Aging and the Nervous System.* Springfield: Charles C Thomas, 1963, pp. 191-216.

23. Schonfield, A.E.D. Learning, memory, and aging. In Birren, J. E., and Sloane, R. B. (eds.), *Handbook of Mental Health and Aging.* Englewood Cliffs, N.J.: Prentice Hall, 1980, pp. 214-244.

24. Drachman, D. A., and Leavitt, J. Memory impairment in the aged: Storage versus retrieval deficit. *J Exp Psychol* 302, 1972.

25. Hulicka, I. M., and Grossman, J. L. Age-group comparisons for the use of mediators in paired-associate learning. *J Gerontol* 22:46, 1967.

26. Walsh, D. A., and Baldwin, M. Age differences in integrated semantic memory. *Dev Psychol* 13:509-514, 1977.

27. Eriksen, C. W., Hamlin, R. M., and Daye, C. Aging adults and rate of memory scan. *Bull Psychon Soc* 1:259-260, 1973.

28. Anders, T. R., Fozard, J. L., and Lillyquist, T. D. Effects of age upon retrieval from short-term memory. *Dev Psychol* 6:214-217, 1972.

29. Kinsbourne, M. Cognitive decline with advancing age: An interpretation. In Smith, W. L., and Kinsbourne, M. (eds.) *Aging and Dementia.* New York: Spectrum, 1977, p. 217.

30. Macht, M. L., and Buschke, H. Cognitive effort in remembering in aging. *J Gerontol,* 1983.

31. Eisdorfer, C., and Wilkie, F. Intellectual changes with advancing age. In Jarvik, L. F., Eisdorfer, C., and Blum, J. E. (eds.), *Intellectual Functioning in Adults.* New York: Springer, 1973, pp. 25-29.

32. Blum, J.E., Clark, E.T., and Jarvik, L.F.: The New York State Psychiatric Institute Study of Aging Twins. In Jarvik, L.F., Eisdorfer, C., and Blum, J.E. (eds.), *Intellectual Functioning in Adults.* New York: Springer, 1973, p. 13.

33. American Psychiatric Association Task Force on Nomenclature and Statistics. *Diagnostic and Statistical Manual of Mental Disorders. 3rd Ed.* Washington, D.C., 1980, p. 494.

34. Katzman, R. The prevalence and malignancy of Alzheimer's disease: A major killer. *Arch Neurol* 33:217-218, 1976.

35. Gruenberg, E. M. A mental health survey of older people. III. *Psychiatr Q Suppl* 34-35:34-75, 1960-61.

36. Nielsenk, J. Geronto-psychiatric period-prevalence investigation in a geographically delimited population. *Acta Psychiat Scand* 38:307-339, 1973.

37. Sluss, T. K., Gruenberg, E. M., and Kramer, M. The use of longitudinal studies in the investigation of risk factors for senile dementia-Alzheimer type. In Mortimer, J. A., and Schuman, L.M. (eds.), *The Epidemiology of Dementia.* New York: Oxford University Press, 1981, pp. 132-154.

38. Hagnell, O., Lanke, J., Rorsman, B., and Ojesjo, L. Does the incidence of age psychosis decrease? *Neuropsychobiology* 7:201-211, 1981.

39. Kral, V. A. Senescent forgetfulness: Benign and malignant. *Can Med Assoc J* 86:257-260, 1962.

40. Blessed, G., Tomlinson, B. E., and Roth, M. The association between quantitative measures of dementia and of senile changes in the cerebral grey matter of elderly subjects. *Br J Psychiatry* 114:797-811, 1968.

41. Haase, G. R. Diseases presenting as dementia. In Wells, C. E. (ed.), *Dementia*. 2nd Ed. Philadelphia: F. A. Davis, 1977. p. 26.

42. Tomlinson, B. E. Morphological changes and dementia in old age. In Smith, W. L., and Kinsbourne, M. (eds.), *Aging and Dementia*. New York: Spectrum, 1977, pp. 25-56.

43. Sourander, P., and Sjogren, H. The concept of Alzheimer's disease and its clinical implications. In Wolstenholme, G.E.W., and O'Connor, M. (eds.), *Alzheimer's Disease and Related Conditions*. CIBA Foundation Symposium. London: J & A Churchill, 1970, p. 11.

44. Jellinger, K. Neuropathological aspects of dementias resulting from abnormal blood and cerebrospinal fluid dynamics. *Acta Neurol Belg* 76:83-102, 1976.

45. Wells, C.E. Diagnostic evaluation and treatment in dementia. In Wells, C.E. (ed.), *Dementia*. 2nd Ed. Philadelphia: F. A. Davis, 1977, p. 247.

46. Tomlinson, B. E., Blessed, G., and Roth, M. Observations on the brains of demented old people. *J Neurol Sci* 11:205-242, 1970.

47. Thomas, L. On the problem of dementia. *Discover*, pp. 434-436, August 1981.

48. Rosenwaike, I., Yaffe, N., and Sagi, P. C. The recent decline in mortality of the extreme aged: An analysis of statistical data. *Am J Public Health* 70:1074, 1980.

49. Katzman, R., Terry, R. D., and Bick, K. L. (eds.). *Aging*, Vol. 7: *Alzheimer's disease: Senile dementia and related disorders*. New York: Raven Press, 1978, p. 1.

50. Alzheimer, A. Ueber eine eigenartige Erkraenkung der Hirnrinde. *Allgemeine Zeitschrift fuer Psychiatrie* 64:146, 1907.

51. Terry, R., and Katzman, R. Senile dementia of the Alzheimer type: Defining a disease. In Katzman, R., and Terry, R. (eds.), *Neurology of Aging*. Philadelphia: F. A. Davis, 1983, pp. 51-84.

52. Terry, R. D., Gonatas, N. K., and Weiss, M. Ultrastructural studies in Alzheimer's presenile dementia. *Am J Pathol* 44:269-297, 1964.

53. Terry, R. D., and Wisniewski, H. M. The ultrastructure of the neurofibrillary tangle and the senile plaque. In Wolstenholme, G.E.W., and O'Connor, M. (eds.), *Alzheimer's Disease and Related Conditions*. CIBA Foundation Symposium. London: J & A Churchill, 1970, p. 145.

54. Wisniewski, H. M., Narang, H. K., Corsellis, J.A.N., and Terry, R. D. Ultrastructural studies of the neuropil and neurofibrillary tangle in Alzheimer's disease and post-traumatic dementia. *J Neuropathol Exp Neurol* 35:367, 1976.

55. Katzman, R., Brown, T., Fuld, P., Peck, A., Schechter, R., and Schimmel, H. Validation of a short Orientation-Memory-Concentration Test of cognitive impairment. *Am J Psychiatry*, 1983.

56. Bowen, D. M., Smith, C. B., White, P., and Davison, A. N. Neurotransmitter-related enzymes and indices of hypoxia in senile dementia and other abiotrophies. *Brain* 99:459-495, 1976.

57. Davies, P., and Maloney, A.J.R. Selective loss of central cholinergic neurons in Alzheimer's disease. *Lancet* II:1403, 1976.

58. Perry, E. K., Perry, R. H., Blessed, G., and Tomlinson, B. E. Necropsy evidence of central cholinergic deficits in senile dementia. *Lancet* I:189, 1977.

59. Davies, P., and Verth, A. H. Regional distribution of muscarinic acetylcholine receptor in normal and Alzheimer's type dementia brains. *Brain Res* 138:385-392, 1977.

60. Drachman, D. A. Memory, dementia, and the cholinergic system. In *Aging*, Vol. 7: *Alzheimer's Disease: Senile Dementia and Related Disorders*. Katzman, R., Terry, R. D., and Bick, K. L. (eds.). New York: Raven Press, 1978, pp. 141-150.

61. Drachman, D. A., and Leavitt, J. Human memory and the cholinergic system. *Arch Neurol* 30:113-121, 1974.

62. Perry, E. K., Tomlinson, B. E., Blessed, G., Bergmann, K., Gibson, P. H., and Perry, R. H. Correlation of cholinergic abnormalities with senile plaques and mental test scores in senile dementia. *Br Med J* 2:1457-1459, 1978.

63. Davies, P., Katzman, R., and Terry, R. D. Reduced somatostatin-like immunoreactivity in cerebral cortex from cases of Alzheimer disease and Alzheimer senile dementia. *Nature* 288:279-280, 1980.

64. Cross, A. J., Crow, T. J., Perry, E. K., Perry, R. H., Blessed, G., and Tomlinson, B. E. Reduced dopamine-beta-hydroxylase activity in Alzheimer's disease. *Br Med J* 282:93-94, 1981.

65. Rossor, M., Fahrenkrug, J., Emson, P., Mountjoy, C., Iversen, L., and Roth, M. Reduced cortical choline acetyltransferase activity in senile dementia of Alzheimer type is not accompanied by changes in vasoactive intestinal polypeptide. *Brain Res* 201:249-253, 1980.

66. Johnston, M. V., McKinney, M., and Coyle, J.T. Evidence for a cholinergic projection to neocortex from neurons in basal forebrain. *Proc Nat Acad Sci USA* 76:5392-5396, 1979.

67. Whitehouse, P. J., Clark, A. W., Price, D. L., Struble, R. G., DeLong, M. R., and Coyle, J. T. Alzheimer's disease: Loss of cholinergic neurons in the nucleus nasalis. *J Neuropathol Exp Neurol* 40:323, 1981.

68. Terry, R. D., Peck, A., DeTeresa, R., Schechter, R., and Horoupian, D. S. Some morphometric aspects of the brain in senile dementia of the Alzheimer type. *Ann Neurol* 10:184-192, 1981.

69. Corsellis, J.A.N. Mental Illness and the Aging Brain. Maudsley Monograph No. 9. London: Oxford University Press, 1962.

70. Frackowiak, R.S.J., Pozzilli, C., Legg, N. J., du Boulay, G. H., Marshall, J., Lenzi, G. L., and Jones, T. Regional cerebral oxygen supply and utilization in dementia. A clinical and physiological study with oxygen-15 and positron tomography. *Brain* 104:753-778, 1981.

71. Thal, L. J., Rosen, W., Sharpless, N. S., and Crystal, H. Choline chloride fails to improve cognition in Alzheimer's disease. *Neurobiol Aging* 2:205-208, 1981.

72. Thal, L. J., Fuld, P. A., Masur, D. M., and Sharpless, N. D. Oral physostigmine and lecithin improve memory in Alzheimer's disease. *Ann Neurol* 13:491-496, 1983.

73. Davis, K. L., Mohs, R. C., Rosen, W. G., Greenwald, B. S., Levy, M. I., and Horvath, T. B. Letter to the Editor. *New Eng J Med* 308:721, 1983.

74. Cook, R. H., Ward, B. E., and Austin, J. H. Studies in aging of the brain: IV. Familial Alzheimer disease: Relation to transmissible dementia, aneuploidy and microtubular defects. *Neurology* 29:1402-1412, 1979.

75. Larsson, T., Sjogreni, T., and Jacobson, G. Senile dementia. *Acta Psychiatr Scand* 39 (Suppl. 167) 3, 1963.

76. Heston, L. L., Mastri, A. R., Anderson, V. E., et al. Dementia of the Alzheimer type: clinical genetics, natural history and associated conditions. *Arch Gen Psychiatry*, 1981.

77. Jarvik, L. F. Genetic factors and chromosomal aberrations in Alzheimer's disease, senile dementia, and related disorders. In Katzman, R., Terry, R., and Bick, K. L. (eds.), *Aging*, Vol. 7: *Alzheimer's Disease: Senile Dementia and Related Dis-*

orders. New York: Raven Press, 1978, pp. 273-278.

78. Cook, R. H., Schneck, S. A., and Clar, D. B. Twins with Alzheimer's disease. *Arch Neurol* 38:300-301, 1981.

79. Burger, P. C., and Vogel, F. S. The development of the pathologic changes of Alzheimer's disease and senile dementia in patients with Down's syndrome. *Am J Pathol* 73:457-476, 1973.

80. Wisniewski, K., et al. Precocious aging and dementia in patients with Down's syndrome. *Biol Psychiatry* 13:619-627, 1978.

81. Yates, C. M., Simpson, J., Maloney, A.F.J., Gordon, A., and Reid, A. H. Alzheimer-like cholinergic deficiency in Down's syndrome. *Lancet* II:979, 1980.

82. Heston, L. L. Alzheimer's disease and senile dementia: Genetic relationships to Down's syndrome and hematologic cancer. In Katzman, R. (ed.), *Congenital and Acquired Cognitive Disorders*. Research Publications of the Association for Research in Nervous and Mental Diseases, Vol. 57. New York: Raven Press, 1979, pp. 167-176.

83. Crapper, D. R., Krishnan, S. S., and Dalton, A. J. Brain aluminum distribution in Alzheimer's disease and experimental neurofibrillary degeneration. *Science* 180:511-513, 1973.

84. Perl, D. P., and Brody, A. R. "Alzheimer's disease: X-Ray spectrometric evidence of aluminum accumulation in neurofibrillary tangle-bearing neurons. *Science* 208:207-209, 1980.

85. Markesbery, W. R., Ehmann, W. D., Hossain, T.I.M., Alauddin, M., and Goodin, D. T. Brain trace element levels in Alzheimer's disease by instrumental neutron activation analysis. *J Neuropathol Exp Neurol* 40:359, 1981.

Informal Social Support Systems for the Frail Elderly

Barbara Silverstone*

In increasing numbers, very old persons are suffering from chronic mental and physical impairments which demand responses from the social environment extending far beyond conventional short-term interventions. These responses may include ongoing medical, rehabilitative, and skilled nursing attention, help with basic daily chores, and assistance with the more complex financial and bureaucratic negotiations of modern life. The provision of these extended arrangements, directly or indirectly, becomes most naturally the responsibility of close family members and, at times, friends. The history of reciprocity and the filial commitments that characterize these relationships undergird such efforts. This paper summarizes what is currently known about the extent and quality of these extended arrangements between frail, impaired elders and their families and friends, the associated burdens and stresses placed upon informal care providers, their expressed needs for help, and the types of programs developed thus far in response. At the same time, gaps in knowledge of the informal support system are identified, and public policy concerns associated with this subject are formulated for study.

*Executive Director, The Lighthouse, New York Association for the Blind, New York, New York.

THE ELDERLY AND THEIR INFORMAL
SOCIAL NETWORKS

Informal supports for the frail elderly must be viewed within the larger context of their social networks. Demographic patterns, family structure, roles and functions, household living arrangements, and socioeconomic status all contribute to the character and quality of long-term care arrangements.

More than a decade has passed since sociologists established the now well-accepted fact that the elderly, although largely segregated from the formal bureaucratic structures of society, are well integrated into the informal social network of families, friends, and neighbors (Shanas et al., 1968). This remains true in spite of the fact that the American family structure has shifted dramatically since the turn of the century, extending in generations due to growing numbers of persons surviving into old age but diminishing within generational cohorts because of decreasing fertility rates. The latter trend is substantiated by the fact that the average family in 1970 had an average of 2.6 children, compared to 4.5 in 1910 (Atchley, 1977). The extension of generations is supported by the fact that 10 percent of those now over the age of 65 have living children also over the age of 65. Seventy percent of the elderly are grandparents and 40 percent, great-grandparents. Seventy percent of those over the age of 70 have living siblings (Shanas, 1979a).

Marriage for elderly men is the most important family relationship. Most males (77 percent) over the age of 65 are married and living with their spouses. However, only 37.8 percent of females over 65 are married and living with their spouses. Over the age of 85, the percentage of married males drops to 33 percent and for females to 8 percent. These figures reflect the longer life expectancy of women and the fact that men tend to marry younger women (Glick, 1979; U.S. Bureau of the Census, 1982a).

Most of the elderly with children see them often or maintain contact by telephone or mail. Eighty percent of those with children report seeing their children at least once a week. Seventy-five percent live within a 30-minute drive of a child (Shanas, 1979b). The affective component between generations appears on the average to be strong, with children often viewed as confidants by their elderly parents (Bengston and Treas, 1980). Interaction with children extends beyond socialization, and for the majority there is a mutual exchange of goods and services although this tends to decrease for elders when frailty or impairment occurs (Troll, 1979).

In spite of the reciprocity between elders and their children, Bengston and Kuypers (1971) stress the different perspectives of each generation. Although the elderly report higher levels of affection in their relationships with children than do the children, they minimize the amount of assistance or exchange of services. Sociologists also stress the mediating role families play for elders, often serving as brokers with bureaucracies and conveyors of the norms to be followed in coping with the crises of old age (Sussman, 1977; Bengston and Treas, 1980).

Contacts with more distant kin, including grandchildren, are far less frequent than with children and some elders report discomfort with the grandparenting role (Hill, 1965). Neugarten and Weinstein (1964) describe different patterns of grandparenting, ranging from being friend to sage. Lopata (1975) found that, except for children, kin were not highly supportive in the lives of widows. Racial and ethnic variations exist, however; and Kulys and Tobin (1980) cite greater cooperative involvement with extended family and friends among blacks than among whites.

Friendships are also important to the elderly. In a national survey, Louis Harris and Associates (1975) found that the most popular activity of the elders interviewed was "socializing with friends." Loneliness was reported as a serious problem by only 12 percent of those 65 and over. Maddox (1968), however, notes that there does appear to be a general decrease in activity levels at very old age, perhaps because of frailty and loss of friends. As with families, friends are cited as confidants by elders and play an important role in providing affective support (Rosow, 1967). In all, social isolation is not a prevalent condition for elders (Silverstone and Miller, 1980).

Although relationships with family and friends are reported to be satisfactory to elders for the most part, they tend to live apart as married couples or alone, but close to their children (Shanas, 1979a). For the young old, the most typical living arrangement is with a spouse. One in six elderly age 65 and over shares a dwelling with an adult child (Schorr, 1980). The majority of elders do not choose to live with their children, although the possibility increases for both men and women in the very late years, paralleling the increase in institutionalization. Fourteen percent of very old men (85 +) live with a child, as do 26 percent of women (85 +). Over 20 percent of elders age 85 and over live in institutions, as contrasted to 5 percent for the total elderly population. Living with an unrelated adult is rare for the elderly. In general, living alone has become an increasingly common life style for elders as well as for younger adults, particularly marked in the period 1970–1976. Forty-two percent of older women (65 +) and 14 percent of older men are now living alone (Glick, 1979; Brotman, 1982; U.S. Bureau of Census, 1982a).

A positive effect on the family has been the significant economic strides made by the elderly in recent decades as a result of the increasing benefits of Social Security and retirement pensions. Health care insurance (Medicare), although far from equitable or comprehensive in coverage, particularly in relation to long-term care, is another financial bulwark for the elderly. As a result, the financial burden on children in the postwar decades has been negligible, with only 9 percent of the elderly receiving regular financial help from their children and only 3 to 4 percent, occasional help (Troll, 1979). This dramatic decrease in financial dependence between the generations, in the opinion of some experts, accounts for the abundance of social and affective exchanges (Treas, 1977).

Nevertheless, the elderly remain the poorest age group. In 1979, one-fourth of the 65 + population were classified as poor or near-poor. Elders living alone, who most often are women, tend to be poorer. Sixty-eight percent of those elderly living alone received incomes of less than $6,000 in 1968 compared to 46 percent of the total population living alone. Members of minority groups are significantly over-represented in the ranks of the elderly poor, with the poverty rate for older black women reaching 42 percent in 1979, contrasted to 16 percent for older white women (Federal Council on the Aging, 1981; White House Conference, 1981).

In summary, a rich fabric of informal relationships envelops the majority of elders in our society along a number of dimensions. This fabric is bonded most strongly by marriage and adjacent generational and peer relationships and, for racial minorities, by extended kin as well. The stake elders maintain in these informal relationships extends beyond dependence for services, with social contacts and affectional and material exchanges far greater between generations than commonly believed. While elders tend to live alone or with a spouse, they are generally not socially isolated and are part of an extended family network. This aggregate portrayal, however, belies marked differences for subpopulations of the elderly. Women tend to be more isolated, and as elders move into very old age the informal structure diminishes considerably for both sexes, particularly in relation to marriage and peer relationships. Other critical contrasts will surface in considering informal supports vis-à-vis long-term care.

INFORMAL SUPPORTS AS PROVIDERS OF LONG-TERM CARE

The sturdiness that characterizes the informal social networks of the elderly is reflected in the care and support given them when illness occurs. A national sample of older persons indicated that, in a health crisis, 80 to 90 percent of elders with adult children would seek assistance from them if help was needed (Shanas et al., 1968). Over 80 percent of all home care is actually provided to impaired elders by family members, supporting the fact that the elderly generally turn to family members for help and for the most part receive it (U.S. National Center for Health Statistics, 1975).

A 1977 study by the General Accounting Office (GAO) of a random sample of 1,609 elderly in Cleveland found that although 23 percent were assessed as impaired, 56 percent were actually receiving help from family or friends. The most frequently provided services were transportation (60 percent) and checking on the elder's well-being (44 percent). Next in order of frequency were homemaker services (20 percent), administrative and legal assistance (15 percent), meal preparation (13 percent), housing (12 percent), and coordination (8 percent). Groceries and food stamps (7 percent), continuous supervision (6 percent), nursing care (3 percent), and general financial aid (2 percent) were the least-provided services (U.S. General Accounting Office, 1977a,b; Tobin and Kulys, 1980).

In this same study, family care was costed out and found to exceed the cost or value of services provided by agencies at all levels of impairment. For the extremely impaired, the cost or value of services provided by family and friends averaged $673 per month as contrasted with $172 for services provided by agencies (U.S. General Accounting Office, 1977b).

While some studies find adult children the most frequent source of help to elders (U.S. General Accounting Office, 1977a,b), others suggest that it is the spouse who is the most frequent source of help (Shanas, 1979b). This discrepancy is probably explained by the marital status of the elder, the type of help sought, and the condition of the spouse. Friends and neighbors appear more often to deliver intermittent, supplementary assistance and are less able than the family to cope with impaired and disabled individuals on a long-term basis (Litman, 1971; Shanas and Maddox, 1976; Shanas, 1979b). Cantor (1980) underscores the fact that friends and neighbors occupy a position of secondary support to children. However, they become considerably more important for older persons who have no kin.

The adult daughter has been frequently cited as an important source of family help. Brody (1979) interviewed 161 three-generation families—grandmothers, daughters, and granddaughters—to determine the amount and nature of help that middle-aged daughters provide to elderly mothers and the relationship between the daughter's care-giving activities and other characteristics. Overall, daughters with a mean age of 49 provided help to their mothers an average of 8.6 hours per week, increasing to 28.5 hours per week if the mother lived in the home. Daughters in their 50s and older provided more than 15 hours per week.

In another study, Horowitz (1981) found that some sons assumed the care-giver role by default, primarily because no daughter was available. There were no gender differences in number of contacts with the parents or the degree of emotional support, but it was found that generally daughters were significantly more likely to help parents in the areas of hands-on assistance. When it became necessary, some daughters-in-law provided direct care to parents-in-law as well as providing support to their husbands.

Secondary analysis of the data collected for the GAO study of Cleveland elderly (1977b) found no differences by age, race, or education and expectations for receiving help from others, but differences were found by age, race, and socioeconomic status with regard to the source of help to the elder, the younger elder more frequently citing spouses and siblings and the older aged citing children and friends. Extended kin and friends were mentioned more often by black respondents, while spouses were more often mentioned by respondents in a higher socioeconomic category. The greater use of formal support among the higher socioeconomic groups may have been due to smaller kin groups and greater financial resources, but the overall expectation among the aged was for long-term assistance from nuclear kin, regardless of age, race, or socioeconomic status (Noelker, 1980). In general, socioeconomic status has been found to be a more useful variable than race and ethnicity in explaining differences in family support (Seelbach, 1978).

There seems to be little question that elders have clear preferences regarding sources of support, with family being most important and formal organizations important when family is not available. The mitigating effects of informal supports on the risk of institutionalization extend beyond tangible services. In their seminal research on confidants, Lowenthal and Haven (1968) found that the presence of a confidant insulated the elderly from institutionalization for mental impairment. A study by Schooler (1975) of 4,000 noninstitutionalized elderly found that having a confidant, particularly a nonfamily member, was highly associated with self-esteem and appeared to reduce the adverse effects of poor environmental conditions. The affective and associational dimensions of informal relations may prove to be as critical in long-term support of the frail elderly as the provision of services.

Strong patterns of family support in relation to general services and intermittent health care, however, may be less impressive when examined in terms of intensity and duration. Cantor (1980) found that formal supports assumed greater importance as age and degree of frailty increase. Forty-three percent of families in a 1971 study indicated difficulty in providing long-term care and 32 percent reported they would be unable to care for a sick person at home under any circumstances (Litman, 1971). In the GAO study of Cleveland elderly, a very small percentage of family assistance involved nursing care and continuous supervision (U.S. General Accounting Office, 1977a,b).

The most intense informal care-giving patterns appear to be found in situations where elders are in residence with families. Brody (1979) found the most extensive help being given by daughters who lived with their mothers. In a study of mentally and physically impaired elders in residence, Poulshock and Noelker (1982) examined 617 families, half of whom were spouse care-givers and half, child care-givers; they found that extensive help was being provided—reportedly for an average of six years. The presence of spouse and children is a critical factor in helping some impaired elders remain in the community. In a sample of nursing home residents and equally impaired community elders, the key variable differentiating the two groups was that the community elders lived with spouse or children (Brody et al., 1978).

Aside from family reports and recollections, these cross-sectional studies tell us little about how kin sustain help over time, particularly when more intense care is required or when family resources are diminished. What is needed are longitudinal studies which follow families over time, as well as studies which carefully differentiate patterns of care-giving, particularly in relation to level of impairment. Just as nursing home rates for the elderly dramatically increase in the later years, so do in-family residence living situations. The question to be answered is how many of the latter are care-giving arrangements for impaired elders.

In summary, family care-giving to impaired elders appears extensive and varied. Spouses and daughters appear to be the primary care-givers, a minor but significant number living with and caring for impaired elders. Other families appear to have serious problems providing extensive and intensive care to the frail elderly. The extent of family care-giving is reflected in the estimated costs, which far exceed those of the formal system. Ethnic and racial differences do not appear to play a great role in differentiating care-giving patterns unless associated with socioeconomic status, where the greater use of formal services is associated with smaller kin networks and greater financial resources. The dearth of longitudinal studies regarding informal supports to the frail elderly needs to be remedied in order to ascertain the actual extent and duration of informal care-giving (particularly in relation to impairment levels), which cross-sectional studies may exaggerate or minimize.

QUALITY OF CARE

Little is known about the quality of care provided by families and friends to impaired frail elders. While it has been documented that elders prefer the help of family, questions remain about the degree of skill which families bring to the care of the moderate to severely impaired elder, as well as the extent of family abuse.

In one of the few in-depth studies to examine these care-giving issues, family members who lived with and cared for their elders reported difficulty in caring for mentally impaired elders, particularly those exhibiting negative behavior (Poulshock and Noelker, 1982). Incontinence and heavy lifting were also problems for the families. While 91 percent of the elders who could be interviewed generally reported few complaints and stated they preferred to continue their present arrangement, 90 percent admitted they were dependent on their care-giver and 55 percent complained that their care-givers did too much for them. Thirty percent agreed that their relationship with their care-giver made them feel useless. One might postulate that this population—as with some nursing home residents—might be experiencing conditions of "excess disability" or functional loss not justified by their actual physical and mental impairments (Lawton and Brody, 1969). The high degree of reported incontinence on the part of the elders (over 50 percent) gives further support to this hypothesis, for such a condition can be exacerbated by improper facilities or nursing and medication regimens. In any case, family care of frail and impaired elders cannot automatically be assumed to be skilled care regardless of the degree of filial responsibility, love, and devotion. These very qualities may in and of themselves promote overprotectiveness and tension.

The issue of exploitative and aggressive behavior between helpless frail elders and their care-givers has long been recognized in nursing homes (Vladeck, 1980). More recently, the focus has broadened to include families and neighbors of elders in the community. Steinmetz (1983) interviewed 77 adult children who were caring for elderly relatives at the time of the interview or who had done so within the past three years. The "abuser" was likely to be a woman in her late 50s or early 60s who had responsibilities to children and grandchildren and also carried responsibility for care of a parent in his or her eighties. Abusive tactics were found to be used as a last resort when other conflict resolution techniques failed. About 10 percent of the elderly had experienced either threats or acts of violence from their children. Eight percent of the children had used physical restraints, 5 percent threatened physical violence, and 1 percent used either hitting, slapping, or shaking. Violence by the elders against their children was also reported, with 18 percent of the parents slapping, hitting, or throwing objects at their care-givers. Other conflict resolution techniques used by some elders included pouting, screaming, and yelling.

Isolated incidences of abuse by family, friends, or neighbors have appeared with increasing frequency, and in some states professionals are required by law to report these situations, which are difficult to document because of the reluctance or inability of elders to complain about their families. Factors considered to contribute to elder abuse include a family pattern of violence, violence associated with drug or alcohol abuse, the inability of family members to tolerate the dependency of an older relative, and stresses associated with caring for and living with an impaired elder (Rathbone-McCuan, 1980). Incidents of family abuse, however, while requiring attention, are considered to be exaggerated by both professionals and the media, who may be perpetuating negative stereotypes about the families of the old.

EFFECTS OF CARE-GIVING ON INFORMAL SUPPORTS

Thus far, it has been established that informal support and care-giving to frail elders is extensive and costly, is provided primarily by spouses and daughters, and is preferred by elders over other forms of long-term care. While normative patterns of intense long-term care-giving arrangements exist, much is still to be learned about the patterns and duration of care-giving in relation to impairment level as well as about the quality of care. But what of the effects on the family itself, which may in turn have an impact on quality of care?

The effects on families of providing care to the frail and impaired elderly are generally assumed to be negative because of the burdens involved. Undoubtedly because of the anticipated burdens, some families opt not to assume the direct care-giving role if there are sufficient funds to purchase services (Cantor, 1980). In a number of instances nursing home placement is sought in advance, but more often only after extended attempts at family care-giving (Brody, 1966).

In addition to their actual physical capacities for care-giving, the degree of stress placed on the family and its ability to manage or tolerate this stress will, to some extent, determine its capacity for ongoing care-giving and the quality of care (Tonti, 1983). The effects also have important implications for other aspects of family functioning, including, among many factors, mental health, the care of children, and economic resources. Knowledge of these effects, therefore, is critical.

In their longitudinal study of family burden in caring for a mentally impaired aged relative, Hoenig and Hamilton (1966) found that 66 percent of the families reported adverse effects on the household as a result of the elder's illness. Primary among these adverse effects were a disruption of family routine and physical strain. Seventy-two percent of the impaired aged in this study demonstrated some type of disturbing behavior which caused additional family problems. The most burdensome problems reported by the families were providing physical or nursing care, followed by the elder's excessive demands for companionship.

Sanford's (1975) research conducted on families of elderly persons who resided in hospital geriatric units in London identified those problems encountered by the family that prevented them from accepting the older person back into their homes. In 50 of these families, the relative who had been the elder's primary care-giver prior to hospital admission was interviewed. The most frequently reported problems, some of which were felt to be "intolerable," included disruptive behavior patterns of the elder, the general immobility of the aged person, personal problems such as anxiety or depression generated by the care-giving role, restrictions on social activities, and a change in environmental conditions because of the presence and needs of the elder.

Isaacs (1971) investigated the reasons why 280 elders were admitted from their homes into a British geriatric unit. In half of these cases, relatives who cared for the aged person had experienced strain to an extent that their physical or mental health was threatened. Findings indicated that excessive strain was frequently the result of the elder's incontinence, immobility, or mental abnormality. Of these three, the most burdensome problem for family members to bear was mental abnormality, a finding also supported by Hoenig and Hamilton (1966).

Review of these studies suggests that mental disturbance in the aged relative is a significant stress-producing factor for other family members. The research of Sainsbury and Grad de Alarcon (1970) lends further support to this finding and goes beyond it by indicating that the mental health of other family members may be affected by the elder's psychiatric disorder. Their study of 119 families with an impaired elderly relative showed that in 63 percent of the cases there were moderate to severe effects on the families' mental health which were related to the family's worry or concern about the elder's behavior.

Lowenthal (1965) reported that exhaustion of a care-giver was second only to unmanageability of the elder as a precipitant to the elder's institutionalization in a psychiatric ward. Archbold (1978) investigated the adult children of aged stroke victims whose stroke had caused loss of function. Findings showed that changes in the care-giver's attitudes and assistance patterns were associated with decrements in the elder's functioning and with the perception that care-giving responsibilities interfered with the care-giver's life style. The majority of these families also evidenced both increased conflict and more illness in the primary care-giver.

Danis (1978) compared the effects of stress among relatives who lived with and cared for an impaired elder with a matched sample of adults without an aged relative in residence. The purpose was to discover which factors, including the elder's morale and severity of the elder's impairment, were associated with the stress experienced by care-givers. Findings showed that a significant source of stress on care-givers was the limitation on their social activities that stemmed from the care-giving burden.

Poulshock and Noelker (1982) found that 617 families caring for impaired elders in residence, usually over extended periods of time, seemed to be coping with their responsibilities. While almost 80 percent of the care-givers reported one or more care-giving tasks as difficult, tiring, or emotionally upsetting, results indicated that the care-givers, on the whole, were not in serious psychological distress. The most commonly reported stressful effect of care-giving was restricted personal time, followed by conflict in the elder–care-giver relationship.

In summary, the research clearly suggests the presence of family stress and dysfunction in relation to taking care of impaired aged relatives, particularly when there are extensive needs for physical or nursing care and when nocturnal disturbances, incontinence, immobility, mental or emotional disturbance, or extensive demands on care-givers are present. Family stress and dysfunction have been manifested by negative changes in family feelings and behavior: anxiety, depression, family conflict, role conflict, and physical illness. Patterns of family care-giving do exist wherein families can function under trying circumstances. What is not known are the contextual variables which account for some families coping with burden and stress and others "giving up." Clues are emerging which suggest that family size, lifestyle, and structure are critical. Zarit et al. (1980) noted that the most important factor that sustained primary family care-givers was help and visitations of other kin. Poulshock (1982) found the strong dyadic relationship between the primary care-giver and elder (usually female spouse and daughter) and secondary supports from other kin were mitigating factors. Race, ethnicity, and socioeconomic status were not factors.

Family epidemiological studies are in order if an accurate picture of care-giving burdens and stress effects is to be drawn. Studies thus far have focused on the tails of the normal curve: the Cleveland study of a selective stratified group of families living with and managing to care for impaired elders, and studies of families with elders in institutions, many of them families who had "given up" because of the burdens and stresses involved. Clearly, both types of families are very real and substantial in number. But a majority of families and other informal supports neither live with nor have placed their elders. The extent, patterns, and quality of their efforts and the effects upon them remain to be identified. Another important quality of care issue relates to family coping patterns, wherein care-giving to the elder is beneficial and family burden and stress are minimal. Knowledge of such coping patterns, now available only by inference, would be indispensable in aiding dysfunctional families.

UNMET NEEDS AND DEMANDS OF FAMILIES AND PROGRAMMATIC RESPONSES

It is generally assumed by gerontologists that respite care, supportive services, and education and training are most needed and wanted by families of chronically impaired elders and that, given these services, families will be better able to sustain care in the community. The planned services of many community agencies are predicated on these assumptions, and there is no question from their experience that they are meeting a need and demand (Safford, 1980; Silverstone and Burack-Weiss, 1983; Zimmer, 1983). The extensive use of nursing homes by families, particularly for the very frail and old, is another case in point. However, these assumptions about unmet needs and demands appear to be based on more basic assumptions, i.e., that a large number of elders are not well cared for and a large number of families are burdened and stressed. As has been noted, a case has yet to be made for proving or disproving either assumption. Furthermore, current utilization rates cannot be used to measure unmet need and demand. Those families who utilize services may be very different from those who do not, problems in access, service delivery, and availability notwithstanding. Agency and nursing home waiting lists are notoriously poor indicators of need, because short waiting lists do not preclude the existence of a high level of need in the community.

The extent and types of unmet needs, therefore, cannot automatically be projected from current research or present utilization patterns. Geographical variations, the differential use of services by families and elders, and other factors compound the issue, calling for research which is epidemiological and longitudinal in character. The picture is further complicated by the fact that, most often, agencies assess the needs of elders and only rarely, the need of the whole family or informal network.

In one of the few studies to directly tap family need and demand, it was found that, of 617 families caring for elders in residence, only 2 percent reported using mental health counseling services, 12 percent received social work counseling, and 2 percent attended a care-giver training or support group. Only 8 percent reported an unmet need for in-home health and personal care, 13 percent had difficulty getting accepted for services, and 17 percent had difficulty obtaining information about available services. Twenty percent complained of their difficulty in getting service providers to come to the home. Financial need was not mentioned. When the primary care-giver did report a need for help in regard to particular tasks, other kin were usually seen as the source of help (Poulshock and Noelker, 1982).

In their study of 29 care-givers for severely mentally impaired elders, Zarit et al. (1980) suggested that unmet need was closely related to the impaired elder's natural support system and that interventions involving informal supports would be helpful. On the other hand, another small study, this one of 30 female care-givers either providing care or managing services, reported their care-giving needs as relief from some care-providing activities:

help in developing management strategies for common problems, and accessible information and referral for service needs (Archbold, 1982).

Clearly, need must be differentiated from demand. Need refers to a general assessment of a problem to be addressed, demand to the expressed wishes of families translated into requests for formal help. Given questions about quality of care raised earlier in this paper, there would appear to be a clear need for training and help for families of the mentally impaired. Family readiness to accept this help beyond the kin network remains to be assessed. More effective utilization of kin resources has emerged as a possible need to which the formal system might respond. But, as noted, the lack of longitudinal and epidemiological family studies obscures our knowledge of need and demand. An extensive controlled longitudinal study of Cleveland families promises valuable findings within several years (Poulshock, 1980).

Programs specifically targeted to families of the frail elderly have been developed in response to specific demands, rather than in response to broad-scale assessments of family need and policy thrusts. These programs are educative, service-oriented, and respite-care–oriented in character. Only a few provide follow-up data. Meltzer et al. (1982) studied two institutional respite programs for care-givers in California and New York and found a positive correlation between a higher level of need and a higher demand for respite services, as well as an unexpectedly high rate of institutionalization (12 percent) of the respite care population within one month of use of respite services. Two possible explanations were offered: (1) use of institutional respite services may have represented one last attempt to avoid institutionalization, or (2) respite may have broken down family barriers to institutionalization.

Programs developed at The Benjamin Rose Institute to serve the frail elderly emphasize helping families to problem-solve more effectively in relation to care-giving and supplementing these efforts when necessary with formal services. Of a total yearly caseload of 1,008 elders in 1982, 379 cases were closed, a majority of whom were able to carry on with informal support. A six-month follow up found the majority of elders and families functioning well (Benjamin Rose Institute, 1983).

One of the better known community efforts, the Community Service Society's Natural Supports Program, included task-centered social casework with care-giving families and community-based support groups for family, friends, and neighbors of the disabled elderly. A primary guideline of this program was to strengthen and enhance the care-giving capacity of the natural supports, rather than act as a substitute for their efforts. Caregivers involved in the program were mostly daughters, spouses, and siblings. The program provided services such as home care, respite care, counseling, escort services, and advocacy. Community-wide educational meetings and small support groups were sponsored to meet concrete service needs (education and skills training) and develop peer support and advocacy skills (Zimmer et al., 1977). Support groups for family members caring for Alzheimer's disease victims have proliferated, mostly supported by local chapters of the Alzheimer's Disease and Related Disorders Association. These groups seem to be very successful in offering emotional support and education to families (Cohen and Eisdorfer, 1982).

Programs for families in nursing homes are also receiving increased attention, in recognition of the fact that the segregation of elders from the community does not weaken kin ties (Silverstone, 1978a; Safford, 1980). Smith and Bengston (1979) found that the emotional quality of family relationships improved following institutionalization, perhaps because the direct burden of care-giving was removed. A number of other community demonstration programs are underway, but not directly targeted to families. Rather, they focus on services to the frail elder that presumably offer respite and supplementation to families. Findings to date suggest that elders receiving home care services are maintained longer in the community and life satisfaction is greater, but not at lower cost than institutionalization. Little is known about the impact on families, although it is presumed they have been helped (U.S. General Accounting Office, 1982).

FUTURE CAPABILITIES OF THE INFORMAL SYSTEM

The current lack of epidemiological and longitudinal data on informal supports for the frail impaired elderly compounds future projections. It is generally acknowledged that predictable shifts in family structure, the role of women, and the advanced educational level of families and elders will have significant impact, but the kind and extent are far from certain.

Population estimates for the next 50 years, at least for the middle aged and aged, are fairly accurate since these individuals are now alive. A slower growth rate for the elderly population is expected between the years 1990 and 2010 with the aging of the relatively small number of cohorts born in the Depression years. With the aging of the postwar baby boom population, the number of aged will mushroom between 2010 and 2030, and then growth will again slow down. From the family perspective, relatively large cohorts of middle-aged children will be available from 1990 to 2010 and then shrink in proportion to the elderly population in the ensuing years because of the lower birthrates in the 1960s and 1970s (Federal Council on the Aging, 1981).

The continuing disproportionate growth in the older population will occur together with declines in the under-18 population (Brotman, 1982). Although it may appear that a thinning family structure and growing numbers of elders will place extra burdens on families in the future, the decline in younger age dependents may free adult resources. The dependency ratio, however, obscures the fact that the growing numbers of elders will be heavily concentrated in the old old group where frailty and impairment are prevalent. Their children, furthermore, will be aging. By the year 2000 the old old will increase by 50 percent. They now constitute one-fourth of the over-65 population, and by the year 2000 they will be one-third (Glick, 1979).

Because of the propensity for women to survive into the very late years, the disproportionate growth in the number of widowed women will continue, resulting in approximately 200 women for every 60 men above the age of 85 by the year 2000. The problems of isolation and poverty, therefore, may increase for women, particularly if the growing rate of single households persists. It is also projected that the proportion of divorced women aged 65 to 75 will double by the year 2000 to 22 percent, exacerbating this situation (Glick, 1979). Group living arrangements for impaired elders without considerable formal supports seem an unlikely development. The increasing divorce rate may also affect family solidarity with younger generations which, in turn, may adversely affect care-giving. However, while older women tend not to remarry, younger persons do, thereby proliferating the family structure, particularly for those elders who maintain contact with divorced in-laws (Glick, 1975).

The issue of women working is of great concern because of the traditional role of the female as care-giver to aging parents. While men 45 to 64 are participating less in the labor force, women are working more, increasing from 39 to 50 percent since 1965 (U.S. Bureau of the Census, 1973). In a three-generational study of women concerning their attitudes on filial responsibility, gender roles, and provision of services, Brody (1979) found the younger generations in favor of men sharing more in care-taking tasks and all generations agreeing that working women should pay others to care for elderly parents. Brody also notes, however, that present generations of working women continue to contribute a great deal to the care of aged parents, and expectations that this care will diminish may be unfounded.

Another facet of the increased employment of women is the positive effect this will have on their financial status, particularly in old age. The projected increased numbers of older widows may not be as financially abject as are present cohorts.

The improved educational level for middle- and old-age generations in the years ahead may strengthen what appears to some to be a weakening informal support system. Only 40 percent of today's elders have a high school education. In 30 years, 78 percent will. Similar educational advances will be seen in middle-aged children. Given the strong relationship between education, socioeconomic status, and health (only 8 percent of the population with a high school education live below the poverty line compared with 33 percent for those with no education), there may be a decrease in poor health for the elderly and middle-aged (Federal Council on the Aging, 1981). Elders and families may be better informed consumers, able to organize themselves and demand and purchase formal services, as the affluent do today.

In summary, the gerontological imperative which is upon us, with variations and fluctuations, will become even more compelling in the twenty-first century. Predictions about family size and structure are fairly accurate given the fact that the aged and middle-aged of the future are now alive. A thinning of the family structure is inevitable as more and more elders grow very old with fewer children, grandchildren, and great-grandchildren filling the younger generations, which possibly could free some of the resources of middle-age for the old. Given both longevity and divorce rates, there will be more very old widowed and single women. This might suggest that the burden of long-term care will shift more to the formal system. But still unknown are the years of actual frailty that will affect the old. If the very old improve their health and socioeconomic status, duration of frailty may decrease, creating less burden for families. The future of the informal support system in relation to its impaired elders is largely unknown.

POLICY CONSIDERATIONS

Given the sizeable gaps in our knowledge of the extent, quality, and effects of informal care-giving and support, the need and demand for help and service, and uncertainty about future trends, it is little wonder that policy considerations are tentative and contradictory. As far as the family is concerned, these considerations are also oblique. There is no family policy, per se, in the United States, but rather income maintenance, child welfare, health care, social service, aging, and long-term care strategies. Policies that address the problems of the family unit in relation to its young, old, and weak are absent (Kahn and Kamerman, 1978). In addition, there is no defined neighborhood or community policy to extend the informal system. This is not to say that family units are not profoundly affected by present policies. Social Security, an income maintenance strategy directed toward the welfare of the retired elderly, has removed a considerable financial burden from families and, in the opinion of some, has enhanced the quality of filial relations (Bengston and Treas, 1980).

Families are not dismissed as irrelevant in long-term care policy considerations. The role of the family is being vigorously debated and opinions seem divided into two camps, one based on the assumption that a strong informal structure is in place which can be tapped further in support of the frail elderly, and the other on the assumption that the informal structure, particularly the family, has been stretched as far as possible and will only weaken in the future. Neither view correlates with political ideology and sometimes both are expressed simultaneously.

The first viewpoint is reflected in one set of efforts to revive relative responsibility laws and another set of efforts to create financial incentives to encourage family care-giving. Related to these efforts are expressed concerns that an increase in formal services will supplant family efforts.

The issue of fiscal responsibility of adult children (spouses have always been legally required to care for each other) is gaining momentum, particularly in these times of escalating nursing home costs. The Reagan Administration has amended federal regulations which had prohibited the states under Medicare and Medicaid from requiring children to financially support their elderly parents, usually those in nursing homes (Callahan et al., 1980; Aging Services News, 1983). As a result, a number of states are reviving defunct filial responsibility laws which gathered dust over the years because they could not be enforced or were too expensive to enforce. When these laws were first implemented during the 1930s, it was found that they also tended to alienate elders from their children, who could cross state boundaries to avoid their legal responsibility, thus intensifying the problem the laws were intended to ameliorate (Schorr, 1980). Some believe that such laws contributed to the cycle of poverty and dependency (Garrett, 1979–1980). In point of fact, elders and their families pay over 39 percent of nursing home costs (Brotman, 1982). In terms of home care, the average monthly cost to family and friends extends to $675 per month for the very impaired, and family payments constitute 80 percent of total expenditures for long-term care. (U. S. General Accounting Office, 1977b).

The use of financial incentives or tax credits is seen by some as a means of tapping presumed underutilized family resources or sustaining support now in place, but there is little evidence to support such a view. Sussman (1977) studied the importance of service incentives or financial incentives to families, and found that 81 percent of the families would accept older people into their homes under certain circumstances, but incentives would not be a factor in the decision-making process. Nineteen percent would not take an elder in under any conditions and incentives would do nothing to alter their decision. As for tax credits, the U.S. General Accounting Office (1982) has been reluctant to endorse these because of the difficulty in establishing family eligibility. Given that such bureaucratic roadblocks could be overcome, the amount of money which would accrue to families would probably not be sufficient to serve as a realistic incentive. Care-giving and support to elders seem to emanate from long-standing family relationships which the presence or absence of incentives in whatever form cannot alter.

A parallel concern of those who view the informal support system as strong and potentially stronger is that an increase in community services to elders and their families will supplant the family and open the door to skyrocketing costs (U.S. General

Accounting Office, 1982). They believe that the natural disincentives which exist for nursing home care (elders and families generally do not like nursing homes) are not present in home care. The greater use of formal services by families with higher socioeconomic status supports this fear. What is not known, of course, is whether family care is being supplemented in these cases or whether an urgent need on the part of families and elders is being met. It is also not known to what extent families and elders would actually use outside assistance if available.

The second viewpoint expressed in policy deliberations is that care-giving families are overburdened and under considerable stress, and that the structure of the family is such that nothing further can be expected in the way of support to frail elders now and especially in the future. The changing role of women, higher divorce rates, and a growing very old population are used to support this position, as well as the prediction that the number of nursing home beds in the nation will double in the next decade (Federal Council on the Aging, 1981). The only antidote to this development, the argument goes, is to substantially increase the funding of community-based home care services to serve un-related elders and offer respite to families (Schorr, 1980). Temporary nursing home beds and day programs are frequently mentioned in this context. Furthermore, it is pointed out, demand for all of these formal services will increase with better educated, more affluent older consumers.

A third cluster of policy concerns centers on the redress of current policies and programs which serve as disincentives to family care-giving. One issue addresses the disproportionate funds spent on nursing home care compared to home care. Despite a strong disinclination to use nursing homes, there are strong incentives for elders and families to do so. Public support is far easier to obtain within the nursing home setting than in the community. In fact, elders on Supplemental Security Income are penalized if they live with or receive cash benefits from families. Furthermore, the spend-down features of Medicaid can render an elder and his or her spouse penniless, thus unable to resume life in the community. If the family is unable or unwilling to provide total care, the only choice may be nursing home placement, since care in the community is often not present or available (Kaufman, 1980). Rules for couples receiving Medicaid but not Supplemental Security Income require a similar reduction in income. Not only must the noninstitutionalized spouse manage on less money, but the possible return of the institutionalized spouse to his or her home is in jeopardy because of lack of funds (Federal Council on the Aging, 1981).

COMMENTS

Most probably, each of the policy perspectives and concerns expressed represents a particular aspect of reality. Some families may be able to provide more care, but training and counseling will probably be necessary if family stress and quality of care issues are taken into consideration. Other families will provide for their own kin regardless of inducements from the formal system. There are those who will "give up" if services are more available. Undoubtedly, there are many marginal situations where services, training, and respite indeed make a difference for elder and family. What is clear is that policy initiatives in regard to restoring fiscal responsibility and providing financial incentives are probably impractical and may even be destructive.

In this observer's opinion, varied and imaginative types of partnerships are required between the formal and informal systems, developed on the community level, wherein support and care-giving programs are tailored to meet local needs. If a family policy can indeed be devised, it would focus on an assessment of the strengths and incapacities of the family as well as those of the elder, and take into account all the responsibilities facing a family. Family and friends would perform those tasks most suitable to their skills and capacities. Their role as confidant would be as valued as their service contributions, since this role may be just as important as concrete services in sustaining elders in the community. Assistance in family problem-solving and reorganization of family resources would be provided. Formal services would seek to bolster family capacities and supplement them when necessary. Early intervention and prevention would be essential.

However, dynamic community programs (including volunteer services) which interface with the informal system require skilled staff with organizational back-up. Few community agencies in this nation have the capital resources to develop their services flexibly and imaginatively and, when their programs are carried out on a demonstration basis, these agencies lack ongoing funding (Home Care Association of New York State, 1982). Given the severe constraints on resources, the diversion of funding from nursing home expenditures to community programs is required if this is to be a reality (Vladeck, 1980).

Besides needing to correct this unfortunate imbalance between community and institutional services and remove other disin-centives to family care-giving, policy initiatives in long-term care need to be carefully thought out vis-à-vis their impact on the family. As Somers (1980) has noted, the slowing down in the growth rate of the elderly population in the next two decades offers respite to planners. The first order of business is to fill serious knowledge gaps about the informal system and its po-tential. The headlong plunge into nursing home construction and reimbursement in the 1960s and 1970s, while probably helpful to many families, also hurt others, for it misread the needs of those who eschew institutionalization. Sophisticated case man-agement systems now being put into place may also miss the mark in terms of the needs of the informal support system.

SUMMARY

A recurrent theme of this review has been the present dearth of knowledge about informal networks in relation to their support of and care-giving to the frail impaired elderly. Undoubtedly, informal supports, especially the family, are critical to the sur-vival of many elderly in the community, given the gaps in com-munity services and reasonably well-documented knowledge about the larger context of informal relationships. It is also clear that varied normative patterns of informal supports do exist, ranging from intensive in-residence care to affective relationships with-out intensive care-giving services. But the quality of life for im-paired elders over time is not known, nor are the long-range effects on families. Little is known about the strengths and skills of families who do manage well, knowledge which could be tapped for helping other families. Policy considerations are presently limited by this lack of knowledge, although it is very clear that some redress is required in terms of enhancing community ser-vices which, in the opinion of this author, must interface directly with the informal network in a complementary and flexible man-ner. The slower rate of growth of the elderly population in the next two decades offers a much-needed opportunity to correct past mistakes, acquire needed knowledge, and develop sound policies which reflect an accurate appraisal of the frail elder's informal support system.

BIBLIOGRAPHY AND REFERENCES

Aging Services News. States given OK to pass Medicaid familial responsibility laws. April 20, 1983.

Ames, B. D. Care of aging parents by adult offspring. Paper presented at the 35th Annual Scientific Meeting of the Gerontological Society, Boston, November 1982.

Archbold, P. G. Impact of caring for an ill elderly parent on the middle-aged or elderly offspring caregiver. Paper presented at the 31st Annual Meeting of the Gerontological Society, Dallas, November 1978.

Archbold, P. G. All-consuming activity: The family as care-giver. *Generations* VII, 2:12, 1982.

Atchley, R. C. *The Social Forces in Later Life.* 2nd Ed. Belmont, Calif.: Wadsworth, 1977.

Barney, J. L. The prerogative of choice in long-term care. *The Gerontologist* 17:309, 1977.

Baumhover, L. A., and Meherg, J. D. Intergenerational helping patterns: Who cares? Paper presented at the 35th Annual Scientific Meeting of the Gerontological Society, Boston, November 1982.

Bengston, V. L., and Kuypers, J. A. Generational differences and the developmental stake. *Aging and Human Development* 2:249, 1971.

Bengston, V. L., and Treas, J. The changing family context of mental health and aging. In Birren, J. E., and Sloane, R. B. (eds.), *Handbook of Mental Health and Aging.* Englewood Cliffs: Prentice-Hall, 1980, pp. 400-428.

Benjamin Rose Institute. *Quarterly Report of Costs and Services,* January–March, 1983. Cleveland: Benjamin Rose Institute, June 1983.

Bergmann, K., Foster, E. M., Justice, A. W., and Matthews, V. Management of the demented elderly patient in the community. *British Journal of Psychiatry* 132:441, 1978.

Brody, E. M. Women's changing roles, and care of the aging family. In *Aging: Agenda for the Eighties—A National Journal Issues Book.* Washington, D.C.: Government Research Corporation, 1979.

Brody, E. M., and Spark, G. M. Institutionalization of the aged: A family crisis. *Family Process* 5:76, 1966.

Brody, S. J., Poulshock, S. W., and Maschiocchi, C. F. The family caring unit: A major consideration in the long-term support system. *The Gerontologist* 18:556, 1978.

Brotman, H. D. *Every Ninth American.* Washington, D.C.: U.S. Government Printing Office, 1982.

Butler, R. N., and Lewis, M. I. *Aging and Mental Health.* 3rd Ed. St. Louis: Mosby, 1982.

Callahan, D. Supporting parents. *New York Times,* April 11, 1983.

Callahan, J. J., Jr., Diamond, L. D., Giele, J. Z., and Morris, R. Responsibility of families for their severely impaired elders. *Health Care Financing Review* 1:29, 1980.

Cantor, M. H. Neighbors and friends: An overlooked resource in the informal support system. *Research on Aging* 1:435, 1979.

Cantor, M. H. The informal support system: its relevance in the lives of the elderly. In Borgatta, E. F., and McClusky, N. G. (eds.), *Aging and Society: Current Research and Policy Implications.* Beverly Hills: Sage Publications, 1980, pp. 131-144.

Cantor, M. H. The extent and intensity of the informal support system among New York's inner city elderly—Is ethnicity a factor? In *Strengthening Informal Supports for the Aging: Theory, Practice, and Policy Implications.* New York: Community Service Society, 1981a.

Cantor, M. H. Factors associated with strain among family, friends and neighbors caring for the frail elderly. Paper presented at the 34th Annual Meeting of the Gerontological Society, Toronto, November 1981(b).

Cohen, D., and Eisdorfer, C. *Family Handbook on Alzheimer's Disease.* New York: Health Advancement Services, 1982.

Danis, B. G. Stress in individuals caring for ill elderly relatives. Paper presented at the 31st Annual Meeting of the Gerontological Society, Dallas, November 1978.

Danis, B. G., and Silverstone, B. The impact of care-giving: A difference between wives and daughters? Paper presented at the 34th Annual Meeting of the Gerontological Society, Toronto, 1981.

Dobrof, R., and Litwak, E. *Maintenance of Family Ties of Long-Term Care Patients: Theory and Guide to Practice.* Washington, D.C.: U.S. Department of Health, Education and Welfare, 1977.

Dunlop, B. D. Expanded home-based care for the impaired elderly: Solution or pipedream? *American Journal of Public Health* 70:514, 1980.

Federal Council on the Aging. *The Need for Long-Term Care: Information and Issues.* Washington, D.C., 1981.

Frankfather, D. L., Smith, M. J., Caro, F. G. *Family Care of the Elderly: Public Initiatives and Private Obligations.* Lexington, Mass.: D.C. Heath, 1981.

Fries, J. F., and Crapo, L. M. *Vitality and Aging.* San Francisco: W.H. Freeman, 1981.

Garland, B., et al. Personal time dependency in the elderly of New York City: Findings from the U.S.–U.K. Cross-National Geriatric Community Study. In *Dependency in the Elderly of New York City: Policy and Service Implications of the U.S.–U.K. Cross-National Geriatric Community Study.* New York: Community Council of Greater New York, 1978.

Garrett, W. W. Filial responsibility laws. *Journal of Family Law* 18:793, 1979-1980.

Glick, P. C. A demographer looks at American families. *Journal of Marriage and the Family* 37:15, 1975.

Glick, P. C. The future marital status and living arrangements of the elderly. *The Gerontologist* 19:301, 1979.

Hendricks, J., and Hendricks, C. D. *Aging in Mass Society*, 2nd Ed. Cambridge, Mass.: Winthrop, 1981.

Heuser, R. L. *Fertility Tables for Birth Cohorts by Color: United States, 1917–1973.* Rockville, Md: Department of Health, Education and Welfare, National Center for Health Statistics, 1976.

Hill, R. Decision making and the family life cycle. In Shanas, E., and Strieb, G. F. (eds.), *Social Structure and the Family: Generational Relations.* Englewood Cliffs, NJ: Prentice-Hall, 1965.

Hoenig, J., and Hamilton, M. Elderly psychiatric patients and the burden on the household. *Psychiatria et Neurologia*, 152-281, 1966.

Home Care Association of New York State, Inc. *Public Policy for Home Care Development.* Report of Conference on Public Policy for Home Care Development in New York State, October 26–28, 1982.

Horowitz, A. Sons and daughters as caregivers to older parents: Differences in role performance and consequences. Paper presented at the 34th Annual Meeting of the Gerontological Society, Toronto, November 1981.

Howells, D. Reallocating institutional resources: Respite care as a supplement to family care of the elderly. Paper presented at the 33rd Annual Meeting of the Gerontological Society, San Diego, November 1980.

Hudis, I. E., and Buchsbaum, M. D. Components of community-based group programs for family caregivers of the aging. In *Strengthening Informal Supports for the Aging: Theory, Practice, and Policy Implications*. New York: Community Service Society, 1981, pp. 35-43.

Isaacs, B. Geriatric patients: Do their families care? *British Medical Journal* 4:282, 1971.

Johnson, C. L., and Catalano, D. J. A longitudinal study of family supports to impaired elderly. Revision of paper presented at the 35th Annual Meeting of the Gerontological Society, Boston, November 1982.

Kahn, A. J., and Kamerman, S. B. The course of "personal social services." *Public Welfare* 36:29, 1978.

Kaufman, A. Social policy and long-term care of the aged. *Social Work*, 25:133, 1980.

Kobrin, F. E. The fall of household size and the rise of the primary individual in the United States. *Demography*, 13:127, 1976.

Kulys, R., and Tobin, S. S. Older people and their "responsible others." *Social Work* 25:138, 1980.

Lang, A. M., and Brody, E. M. Characteristics of middle-aged daughters and help to their elderly mothers. *Journal of Marriage and the Family* 45:193, 1983.

Lawton, M. P., and Brody, E. M. Assessment of older people: Self-maintaining and instrumental activities of daily living. *The Gerontologist* 9:197, 1969.

Litman, T. J. Health care and the family: A three generational analysis. *Medical Care* 9:67, 1971.

Lopata, H. Z. Support system of elderly urbanites: Chicago of the 1970s. *The Gerontologist* 15:35, 1975.

Louis Harris and Associates, Inc. *The Myth and Reality of Aging in America*. Washington, D.C.: National Council on the Aging, 1975.

Lowenthal, M. F. Social isolation and mental illness in old age. *American Sociological Review*, 12:245, 1965.

Lowenthal, M. F, and Haven, C. Interaction and adaptation: Intimacy as a critical variable. *American Sociological Review* 33:20, 1968.

Lowenthal, M. F., and Robinson, B. Social networks and isolation. In Binstock, R. M., and Shanas, E. (eds.), *Handbook of Aging and the Social Sciences*. New York: Van Nostrand Reinhold, 1976, pp. 432-450.

Lowenthal, M. F., and Simon, A. Mental crises and institutionalization among the aged. *Journal of Geriatric Psychiatry* 4:163, 1971.

Luppens, J., and Lau, E. E. The mentally and physically impaired elderly relative: Consequences for family care. In Kosberg, J. I. (ed.), *Abuse and Maltreatment of the Elderly: Causes and Interventions*. Boston: John Wright, 1983, pp. 204-219.

Maddox, G. L. Persistence of life style among the elderly: A longitudinal study of patterns of social activity in relation to life satisfaction. In Neugarten, B. L. (ed.), *Middle Age and Aging*. Chicago: University of Chicago Press, 1968, pp. 181-183.

Meltzer, J. W. *Respite Care: An Emerging Family Support Service*. Washington, D.C.: The Center for the Study of Social Policy, 1982.

Montgomery, J. E. The economics of supportive services for families with disabled and aging members. *Family Relations* 31:19, 1982.

Montgomery, R.J.V. Impact of institutional care policies on family integration. *The Gerontologist*, 22:54, 1982.

Morgan, L. A. Dual dependencies: Family responsibilities of retirement age males, 1971-1975. Paper presented at the 34th Annual Meeting of the Gerontological Society, Toronto, 1981.

Moroney, R. M. *The Family and the State: Considerations for Social Policy.* New York: Longman Group, 1976.

Morris, R., and Youket, P. The long-term care issues: Identifying the problems and potential solutions. In Callahan, J. J., and Wallace, S. S., *Reforming the Long-Term Care System.* Lexington, Mass.: Lexington Books, 1981.

Neugarten, B., and Weinstein, K. The changing American grandparent. *Journal of Marriage and the Family* 26:199, 1964.

Noelker, L. S. Social resources and use of informal supports: Difference by age, race, and SES. Paper presented at the 33rd Annual Meeting of the Gerontological Society, San Diego, November 1980.

Parsons, T., and Fox, R. Illness, therapy and the modern American family. *Journal of Social Issues* 8:31, 1952.

Poulshock, S. W. *Caring for Elders and the Mental Health of Family Members.* Proposal to the National Institute of Mental Health. Cleveland: Benjamin Rose Institute, 1980.

Poulshock, S. W., and Deimling, G. T. A survey of families caring for elderly: Focus on stress effects. Paper presented at Annual Meeting of the American Orthopsychiatric Association, San Francisco, April 1982.

Poulshock, S. W., and Noelker, L. S. The effects on families of caring for impaired elderly in residence. *Final Report to the Administration on Aging*, 1982.

Prager, E. Subsidized family care of the aged: U.S. Senate Bill 1161. *Policy Analysis* 4:477, 1978.

Preston, S. H., Keyfitz, N., and Schoen, R. *Causes of Death: Life Tables for National Populations.* New York: Seminar Press, 1972.

Rathbone-McCuan, E. Elderly victims of family violence and neglect. *Social Casework* 61:296, 1980.

Rosow, I. *Social Integration of the Aged.* New York: Free Press, 1967.

Safford, F. A program for families of the mentally impaired elderly. *The Gerontologist* 20:565, 1980.

Sainsbury, P., and Grad de Alarcon, J. The effects of community care on the family and the geriatric patient. *Journal of Geriatric Psychiatry* 4:23, 1970.

Sanford, J. R. Tolerance of debility in elderly dependents by supporters at home: Its significance for hospital practice. *British Medical Journal* 3:471, 1975.

Schlesinger, M. R., Tobin, S. S., and Kulys, R. The responsible child and parental well-being. *Journal of Gerontological Social Work* 3:3, 1980.

Schooler, K. Response of the elderly to environment: A stress-theoretical perspective. In Windley, P. G., Byerts, T. O., and Ernst, F. G. (eds.), *Theory Development in Environment and Aging.* Washington, D.C.: Gerontological Society, May 1975, pp. 157-175.

Schorr, A. . . . *Thy Father and Thy Mother* . . . Washington, D.C.: U.S. Department of Health and Human Services, 1980.

Seelbach, W. C. Correlates of aged parents' filial responsibility expectations and realizations. *The Family Coordinator* 7:341, 1978.

Senior Citizen News. New federal policy on Medicaid shifts burden of care to families. May 1983.

Shanas, E. The family as a social support system in old age. *The Gerontologist* 19:169, 1979a.

Shanas, E. Social myth as hypothesis: The case of the family relations of old people. *The Gerontologist*, 19:3, 1979b.

Shanas, E., and Maddox, G. Aging, health, and the organization of health resources. In Binstock, R., and Shanas, E. (eds.), *Handbook of Aging and the Social Sciences.* New York: Van Nostrand Reinhold, 1976, pp. 592-618.

Shanas, E., and Sussman, M. B. (eds.). *Family, Bureaucracy and the Elderly.* Durham, N.C.: Duke University Press, 1977.

Shanas, E., Townsend, P., Wedderburn, D., Henning, F., Milhoj, P., and Stehouwer. *Old People in Three Industrial Societies.* New York: Atherton Press, 1968; reprint ed., New York: Arno Press, 1980.

Sherman, R. H., Horowitz, A., and Durmaskin, S. C. Role overload or role management: The relationship between work and caregiving among daughters of aged parents. Paper presented at the 35th Annual Meeting of the Gerontological Society, Boston, November 1982.

Silverman, P. C. Mutual help and the elderly widow. *Journal of Geriatric Psychiatry* 8:9, 1975.

Silverstone, B. The family is here to stay. *Journal of Nursing Administration* 8:47, 1978a.

Silverstone, B. Family relationships of the elderly: Problems and implications for helping professionals. *Aged Care and Services Review* 1:1, 1978b.

Silverstone, B., and Burack-Weiss, A: *Social Work Practice with the Frail Elderly and Their Families: The Auxiliary Function Model.* Springfield, Ill.: Charles C Thomas, 1983.

Silverstone, B., and Hyman, H. *You and Your Aging Parent.* Expanded ed. New York: Pantheon, 1982.

Silverstone, B., and Miller, S: Isolation in the aged: Individual dynamics, community and family involvement. *Journal of Geriatric Psychiatry* 13:27, 1980.

Smith, K. S., and Bengston, V. L. Positive consequences of institutionalization: Solidarity between elderly parents and their middle-aged children. *The Gerontologist,* 19:438, 1979.

Snider, E. L. The role of kin in meeting health care needs of the elderly. *Canadian Journal of Sociology* 6:325, 1981.

Somers, A. R. Rethinking health policy for the elderly: A six point program. *Inquiry* 17:3, 1980.

Steinmetz, S. K. Dependency, stress, and violence between middle-aged caregivers and their elderly parents. In Kosberg, J. I. (ed.), *Abuse and Maltreatment of the Elderly: Causes and Interventions.* Boston: John Wright, 1983, pp. 134-149.

Sussman, M. B. The family life of older people. In Binstock, R., and Shanas, E. (eds.), *Handbook of Aging and the Social Sciences.* New York: Van Nostrand Reinhold, 1976, pp. 218-243.

Sussman, M. B. Incentives and family environments for the elderly. *Final Report to Administration on Aging.* February 1977.

Tobin, S. S., and Kulys, R. The family and services. In Eisdorfer, C. (ed.), *Annual Review of Gerontology and Geriatrics.* New York: Springer, 1:370, 1980.

Tonti, M. Working with families. In Silverstone, B., and Burack-Weiss, A. *Social Work Practice with the Elderly and Their Families: The Auxiliary Functional Model.* Springfield, Ill.: Charles C Thomas, 1983.

Treas, J. Family support systems for the aged: Some social and demographic considerations. *The Gerontologist* 17:486, 1977.

Troll, L. E., Miller, S. J., Atchley, R. C. *Families in Later Life.* Belmont, Calif.: Wadsworth, 1979, pp. 83-107.

U.S. Bureau of the Census. Census of Population: 1970. Subject Reports, Final Report, Series PC(2)-6A: *Employment Status and Work Experience.* Washington, D.C.: U.S. Government Printing Office, 1973.

U.S. Bureau of the Census. *Current Population Reports,* Series P-60: Characteristics of the Population Below the Poverty Level: 1978. Washington, D.C.: U.S. Government Printing Office, 1980.

U.S. Bureau of the Census. Current Populations Reports, Series P-20, No. 371: *Household and Family Characteristics: March 1981*. Washington, D.C.: U.S. Government Printing Office, 1982a.

U.S. Bureau of the Census. *Statistical Abstract of the United States: 1982-83*. 103rd Ed. Washington, D.C.: Government Printing Office, 1982b.

U.S. Department of Health, Education and Welfare. Public Policy and the Frail Elderly. Washington, D.C.: Federal Council on Aging, 1978.

U.S. General Accounting Office. Comptroller General of the United States. Report to the Congress: Home Health—the Need for a National Policy to Better Provide for the Elderly. Washington, D.C., 1977a.

U.S. General Accounting Office. Comptroller General of the United States. Report to the Congress: The Well-Being of Older People in Cleveland, Ohio. Washington, D.C., 1977b.

U.S. General Accounting Office. Comptroller General of the United States. Report to the Congress of the United States—Conditions of Older People: National Information System Needed. Washington, D.C., 1979.

U.S. General Accounting Office: Report to the Chairman of the Committee on Labor and Human Resources, United States Senate. The Elderly Should Benefit from Expanded Home Health Care but Increasing These Services Will Not Ensure Cost Reductions. Washington, D.C., 1982.

U.S. National Center for Health Statistics. *Vital Statistics of the United States, 1973 Life Tables*. Rockville, Md.: Department of Health, Education and Welfare, 1975.

U.S. National Center for Health Statistics. The National Nursing Home Survey. *Vital and Health Statistics*, Series 13, No. 43, Rockville, Md.: Department of Health, Education and Welfare, 1979.

Vinick B. Elderly men as caretakers of wives. Paper presented at the 35th Annual Meeting of the Gerontological Society, Boston, November 1982.

Vladeck, B. C. *Unloving Care*. New York: Basic Books, 1980.

White House Conference on Aging. *Chartbook on Aging in America*. Washington, D.C.: U.S. Government Printing Office, 1981.

Zarit, S. H., Reever, K. E., and Bach-Peterson, J. Relatives of the impaired elderly: Correlates of feelings of burden. *The Gerontologist* 20:649, 1980.

Zimmer, A. H. Community care for the aged: The natural supports program. In Getzel, G. S., and Mellor, M. J. (eds.), *Gerontological Social Work Practice in Long-Term Care*. New York: Haworth Press, 1983, pp. 149-156.

Zimmer, A. H., Gross-Andrew, S., and Frankfather, D. Incentives to families caring for disabled elderly: Research and demonstration project to strengthen the natural supports system. Paper presented at the 30th Annual Scientific Meeting of the Gerontological Society, San Francisco, November 1977.

Financing Long-term Care for the Elderly:
Institutions, Incentives, Issues

Anne R. Somers*

There is no universally accepted definition of good long-term care (LTC). Agreement on such a definition is one of the urgent tasks facing the Committee on an Aging Society.† For the purpose of this paper, the term is used to refer to services required to improve or maintain the health and functioning of elderly patients with chronic disease and disability, involving significant functional impairment, or to permit death to occur as painlessly as possible. *The goal of such care should always be the maximum functional independence of which the patient is capable.*

The patient's needs may include episodes of acute illness, sometimes requiring hospitalization, but the primary continuing need is for less intensive care, generally lasting at least six months,

---

This paper was prepared for National Academy of Sciences, Institute of Medicine, Committee on an Aging Society, July 1983.

*Adjunct Professor, Department of Environmental and Community Medicine, University of Medicine and Dentistry of New Jersey—Rutgers Medical School, New Brunswick, New Jersey; Lecturer, Woodrow Wilson School of Public and International Affairs, Princeton University, Princeton, New Jersey.

†In keeping with committee emphasis and practical realities, the discussion focuses on the elderly—defined, conventionally, as those age 65 and over. However, many of the same problems, issues, and options apply to the younger disabled and, to a greater or lesser degree, to the entire "aging society." See, for example, Neugarten, B. L. (ed.), Age or Need? Public Policies for Older People. Beverly Hills, Calif.: Sage Publications, 1982.

sometimes years,* and usually involving a combination of medical and social services.† Both institutional and community- or home-based care are included. Although the focus is on formal care, i.e., care that is paid for in one way or another, there is no intention to depreciate the value of informal or unpaid care. On the contrary, good LTC envisions maximum realistic use of family, neighbors, and other volunteers. Nor does the goal of maximum functional independence imply failure in the care of a dying patient. At times, patient autonomy in the choice of where and how to die may constitute maximum functional independence and hence should be facilitated.

It may be objected that this is the definition of an ideal goal rather than the existing situation. This is true. However, agreement on some goal is essential as a yardstick against which to evaluate the rapidly evolving programs, institutions, and personnel, which constitute the "long-term care industry," and for appraisal of the different financial incentives implicit in different methods of paying for such care.

In sharp contrast to the comprehensive, coordinated system contemplated in the above definition, LTC in the United States is highly fragmented and directed far more to "custodial" than to preventive or rehabilitative care. These characteristics were implicit in its historical development. Although the general concept of LTC has emerged only in the past decade, separate elements have long been present in the U.S. health care scene. These include mental hospitals, institutions for the mentally retarded, tuberculosis and other chronic disease hospitals, portions of the Veterans Administration medical system, domiciliary or "old folks' " homes, and some forms of public health nursing. The common denominator for most of these programs was their gen-

---

*There is no agreement on the definition of "long-term" in LTC. The American Hospital Association defines a "long-term hospital" as one where the average length of stay exceeds 30 days (Table 6). The National Center for Health Statistics defines a "chronic condition" as any condition lasting three months or more or a specific list of conditions—heart disease, cancer, stroke, etc.—regardless of duration (Department of Health and Human Services, National Center for Health Statistics, Publication No. (PHS) 81-1232, 1981, p. 332.) This paper concentrates primarily on conditions requiring at least six months' care.

†Obviously, both physical and mental illness are involved. For a discussion of depression and other psychiatric conditions among the elderly, see other papers in this volume.

eral separation from the mainstream of American medicine: different objectives, different institutions, different types of manpower, different methods of financing, and of course different patients. The general acceptance of these differences was clearly expressed and reinforced in legislative concrete in the Medicare law, prohibiting payment for "custodial" care (Social Security Act, Sec. 1862).

However, the American health care scene is dynamic. No sooner had the Medicare capstone been placed on this professional and financial Iron Curtain between acute and chronic care than efforts began to tear it down. Many state mental institutions were closed or drastically reduced in size. Some short-term patients were admitted to community hospitals where they could qualify for Medicare or private insurance. Many patients needing LTC were simply dumped on the community or transferred to nursing homes and Medicaid support. Tuberculosis hospitals were closed or transformed into institutions for general chronic disease with some hope of obtaining Medicare, or at least Medicaid, reimbursement. Even the tightly closed Veterans Administration system began to contract out with some community services.

However, the major assault on the whole hopeless, incurable, "custodial" approach grew out of the "geriatric imperative," with its insistent demand for better and more relevant long-term care.[1] Among the major factors involved in this change of public and professional interest were the increasing life expectancy of the elderly, the growing proportion of elderly in the population, the shift from acute to chronic disease and disability as the major causes of morbidity, the "shrinking" American family and reduced sources of informal LTC, and the escalating costs of all types of health care, especially for the elderly.

By the early 1980s, the demand for reform of LTC had become one of the major health concerns of the nation, probably second only to cost controls. The problem was made doubly difficult, however, by the vastly changed economic and political environment. Whereas the great expansion of funding and other resources for acute care came during the period of unprecedented affluence following World War II, the need for LTC emerged in a period of drastic financial retrenchment. New benefits, which might have been added almost automatically to Medicare, Medicaid, or private health insurance in the 1960s, are now subjected to intense critical and often hostile scrutiny, especially in financial respects. The whole question of financial incentives, largely ignored in the 1960s, has become a major preoccupation of third party payers and policy-makers. It is now virtually impossible to discuss, let alone enact, any significant reform of LTC benefits or systems without considering the incentives embedded in the financial arrangements.

The purpose of this paper is to help identify some major issues involving LTC financial arrangements and incentives and to suggest areas of needed research in relation to each issue. This is the theme of Part III. Part I summarizes the major elements of the LTC industry today; Part II, the principal financing mechanisms that have helped to create and support this industry. Such information is essential to intelligent discussion of the issues.

I. LONG-TERM CARE INDUSTRY

It is impossible to define the LTC industry with precision. Not only is there no precise definition of LTC but the overall institutional, financial, and personnel parameters are expanding and changing rapidly. There is wide disagreement as to what types of institutions, agencies, and programs should be included. Table 1 (which applies to all age groups, not just the elderly), prepared in the Office of the Inspector General for the Secretary of Health and Human Services, represents one reasonable effort at definition. According to this estimate, in 1980 the industry accounted for some $32 billion of health care expenditures, concentrated in three general sectors: (1) nursing homes, $20.5 billion (63 percent); (2) community-based care (including home health care), $6.5 billion (20 percent); and (3) hospitals, $5.3 billion (17 percent). Assuming this $32 billion total increased by only 15 percent per year, a conservative assumption,* by 1983 the total would be nearly $50 billion.

Nursing Homes

Despite the recency of its development and many continuing inadequacies, the nursing home is the dominant LTC institution

---

*Assuming continuation of the 1979 annual growth rates of 18.3 percent for nursing homes, 12.1 percent for hospitals, and 11.9 percent for other LTC programs, LTC expenditures would have increased at an aggregate rate of about 16 percent per year; thus, costs would double every five years. (Ref. 4.)

TABLE 1   Formal Long-Term Care Expenditures in Hospital Care, Nursing Home Care, and Community-Based Care by Source of Funds, 1980[a] (in millions)

Source	Hospital	Nursing Home	Community-Based	Total
Medicare	$1,568[b]	$20,455	$1,042	
Federal Medicaid	419	5,694	85	
Federal Title XX			809[c]	
Administration on Aging			724[d]	
Veterans Administration	1,562	359	723	
Other federal	104	21	135	
State Medicaid	354	4,788	73	
State Title XX			420	
Other state aid	198		211	
Local government			17	
Insurance	902	129	740	
Business/philanthropy	29	129	162	
Consumers	209	8,869	1,377	
Total	5,345	20,444	6,518	$32,307
Federal	3,653	6,529	3,518	13,700
State/local	552	4,788	721	6,061
Private	1,140	9,127	2,279	12,546

[a]Includes all age groups. Excludes income maintenance, food stamps, and community housing assistance estimated at an additional $16.7 billion for the same long-term care population. Also excludes informal or nonpurchased care by family or friends.
[b]"Backed up" hospital patients awaiting nursing home placement.
[c]Mostly in New York and Massachusetts.
[d]Mostly for nutrition.

SOURCE: Department of Health and Human Services, Office of the Inspector General. Long-Term Care: Service Delivery Assessment. Report to the Secretary, 1981 (unpublished), 2 vols. For detailed explanation of estimates see Vol. II, Technical Report.

in the United States today. An estimated 2.4 million Americans use this service annually.[2] Some 5 percent of the elderly population are residents at any given time; the proportion rises to 10 percent of those 75 +, and to 22 percent of those 85 +.[3] It is estimated that 20 percent of the elderly will spend some time in a nursing home before dying. Both the number and proportion of elderly seeking admission to nursing homes will continue to rise, reflecting not only increasing life expectancy but the "shrinking" American family.[4,5] Americans are notoriously negative about this institution, as they once were and to some extent still are about the acute care hospital. But, like it or not, the nursing home is here to stay.

As late as 1960, nursing home expenditures amounted to only $500 million.[6] By 1981 they had reached $24 billion, nearly 10 percent of all personal health care expenditures,[7] over one-fourth of such expenditures for the elderly,[8] and an estimated 63 percent of LTC expenditures (Table 1). Fifty-seven percent of these huge funds come from public sources, primarily Medicaid, which has been a major factor in the rapid expansion and current characteristics of the nursing home industry. In 1977, the elderly comprised 86 percent of the nursing home population,[3] probably even more today.

Information on this industry is very limited. The most complete data come from the 1977 National Nursing Home Survey conducted by the National Center for Health Statistics and a less complete 1973–1974 survey. Tables 2 and 2A provide comparative data from these two surveys.

Over this brief period the total number of homes increased by 20 percent to about 19,000; the number of beds, by 19 percent to 1.4 million.* Average monthly charges rose 44 percent and total expenditures, 77 percent. The average number of beds per institution continued to rise. However, over 75 percent of homes still had fewer than 100 beds in 1977. There was very little change in the geographic distribution. The North Central states retained the largest share; the smallest percentage of homes was in the northeast and of beds, in the west. There is far more regional variation in nursing home beds than in hospital beds. For example, in 1980, there were only 36 beds for every 1,000 elderly individuals in the South Atlantic states compared to 78 per 1,000

---

*The most recent report from the National Center for Health Statistics, 1980 National Master Facility Inventory, identifies 23,065 "nursing and related care homes," with 1.5 million beds and 1.4 million residents. Several definitional differences between this survey and the National Nursing Home surveys cited above and in Tables 2 and 2A preclude meaningful comparisons. (Sirrocco, A. An Overview of the 1980 National Master Facility Inventory Survey of Nursing and Related Care Homes. Advance Data From Vital and Health Statistics, No. 91. National Center for Health Statistics, Department of Health and Human Services Publication No. (PHS) 83-1250. Hyattsville, Md., 1983.)

TABLE 2 Nursing Homes and Beds, Selected Characteristics, United States, 1973–1974 and 1977[a]

| | Nursing Homes | | | | Nursing Home Beds | | | |
| | 1973–1974 | | 1977 | | 1973–1974 | | 1977 | |
Characteristic	Number	Percent Distribution	Number	Percent Distribution	Number	Percent Distribution	Number	Percent Distribution
Total	15,700	100.0	19,900	100.0	1,177,300	100.0	1,402,400	100.0
Ownership								
Proprietary	11,900	75.4	14,500	76.8	832,300	70.7	971,200	69.3
Nonprofit and government	3,900	24.6	4,400	23.2	345,000	29.3	431,200	30.8
Certification[b]								
Skilled nursing facility	5,300	33.5	3,600	19.2	471,900	40.1	294,000	21.0
Skilled nursing and intermediate care facility	2,400	15.4	4,600	24.2	291,600	24.8	549,400	39.2
Intermediate care facility	4,400	28.1	6,000	31.6	253,200	21.5	391,600	27.9
Not certified	3,600	23.1	4,700	25.0	160,000	13.6	167,400	11.9

No. of beds							
Less than 50 beds	6,400	40.8	8,000	42.3	178,800	15.2	182,900	13.0
50–99 beds	5,500	35.0	5,800	30.8	392,500	33.3	417,800	29.8
100–199 beds	3,200	20.4	4,200	22.3	417,900	35.3	546,400	39.0
200 beds or more	600	3.8	900	4.6	188,000	16.0	255,000	18.2
Geographic region							
Northeast	3,100	19.8	3,900	20.5	250,800	21.3	314,900	22.5
North Central	5,600	35.7	5,900	31.1	408,800	34.7	483,900	34.5
South	4,100	26.1	4,900	26.0	303,700	25.8	381,500	27.2
West	2,900	18.4	4,200	22.4	214,100	18.2	222,100	15.8

NOTE: Numbers are rounded to the nearest hundred. Percentages are calculated on the basis of unrounded figures.

[a] Data based on sample surveys. 1977 surveys included all types of nursing homes; the earlier survey excluded those providing only personal or domiciliary care (no nursing). These 500 facilities and 10,000 beds comprised about 2 percent of the homes and 1 percent of the beds.

[b] Medicare extended care facilities and Medicaid skilled nursing homes from the 1973–1974 survey were considered to be equivalent to Medicare or Medicaid skilled nursing facilities in 1977 for purposes of this comparison.

SOURCES: Department of Health and Human Services, National Center for Health Statistics. Utilization of Nursing Homes U.S.: National Nursing Home Survey, August 1973–April 1974, DHEW Publication No. (HRA)77–1779, and the National Nursing Home Survey: 1977 Summary for the U.S., DHEW Publication No. (PHS)79-1794.

TABLE **2A** Nursing Homes and Beds, Selected Characteristics, United States, 1973–1974 and 1977[a]

Characteristic	1973–1974[b]	1977[b]
Admissions (1,000s)	1,111	1,367
Proprietary	853	1,012
Voluntary	258[c]	252
Government		103
Median length-of-stay since		
current admission (days)	547	597
Proprietary	485	597
Voluntary	751[c]	741
Government		698
Average occupancy rate (%)	86.5	89.0
Full-time equivalent personnel:		
rate/100 beds (%)[d]	37.5	46.2
Proprietary	37.0	43.4
Voluntary	36.1	53.7
Government	41.9	49.7
Average monthly charge by		
ownership	$479	689
Proprietary	489	670
Voluntary	456[c]	747
Government		700
By certification		
Skilled nursing facility only	592	880
Skilled nursing and inter-		
mediate care facility	484	762
Intermediate care facility	376	556
Not certified	329	390
Total expenditures (millions)	$7,217[e]	$12,810

[a]Data based on sample surveys. 1977 survey included all types of nursing homes; the earlier survey excluded those providing only personal or domiciliary care (no nursing). These 500 facilities and 10,000 beds comprised about 2 percent of the homes and 1 percent of the beds.

[b]Data for admissions and occupancy rates are for calendar year preceding survey year.

[c]Data for voluntary and government homes were not segregated in 1973–1974.

[d]Only employees providing direct health-related services to patients.

[e]1973.

SOURCES: Department of Health and Human Services, National Center for Health Statistics. Utilization of Nursing Homes U.S.: National Nursing Home Survey, August 1973–April 1974, DHEW Publication No. (HRA) 77-1779, and The National Nursing Home Survey: 1977 Summary for the U.S., DHEW Publication No. (PHS) 79-1794; also Joan F. Van Nostrand, personal communication, June 29, 1983. Fox, P. D., and Clauser, S. B. Trends in Nursing Home Expenditures, Implications for Aging Policy. Health Care Financing Review 1 (Fall):65-70, 1980.

in the West North Central states. The national average in that year was 55.5 per 1,000.[9]

As of 1977, 77 percent of all homes and about 70 percent of the beds were proprietary, that is, operated for profit. Most of the remainder were private nonprofit; about 5 percent were government-operated, mostly by state and local governments. These proportions did not differ greatly between the two surveys, although the proprietary group rose slightly. The most dramatic change has been the growth of proprietary chain operations.* Today over one-third of all homes are part of chains, many of which operate proprietary homes, or home care programs, or both.

Nursing homes are generally classified according to their Medicare or Medicaid certification as skilled nursing facilities (SNFs), which provide 24-hour skilled nursing care under supervision of a physician, or intermediate care facilities (ICFs), which do not have to provide this level of service and are intended for patients who require less intensive care and only on an intermittent basis.

In 1977, the latest year for which complete certification data are available, 32 percent of the homes were ICFs only; nearly one-fourth were both SNFs and ICFs; 19 percent were SNFs only; and one-fourth had no certification. Medicare will reimburse only for SNFs; Medicaid may pay for either, although the proportion of patients in each type of facility varies enormously by state.

The length-of-stay figures require some explanation. Those shown in Table 2A indicate the median stays of all residents on the given survey dates. If all discharges had been counted, as they were in 1977, the picture is quite different. Then the average stay was only 75 days. This reflects the large number of short, mostly Medicare, stays. Although, in this paper, we are primarily concerned with the long-stay patients—whose average length-of-stay is approaching two years—it is important to remember that nursing homes are also extensively used for short-term recuperative and rehabilitative purposes.[2] The latter function is good for staff morale and other qualitative considerations. Carried too far, of course, it can lead to discrimination against long-term, heavy-care patients. The average stay in a voluntary home is 36 percent longer than in a proprietary institution.

---

*The largest of these chains, with 643 homes, reportedly grossed over $800 million in 1982 and anticipates over $1 billion in 1983. (Nursing homes—a new view. (Adv.) New York Times, August 17, 1983.)

Despite industry expansion, the average occupancy rate is high—nearly 90 percent in 1977—and rising. While private pay patients are usually able to find a nursing home bed without too much difficulty, Medicaid patients may have to wait months, even years—a situation that relates both to occupancy rates and to Medicaid reimbursement rates.

As to quality, one measure is staffing; the situation in this respect is very different from the average hospital. Whereas a community hospital maintains a staff of almost 300 full-time equivalents per 100 beds, the average nursing home has fewer than 50. Not surprisingly, the ratios vary widely according to certification status. For example, the 1977 ratios averaged 52.7 for SNFs, 40.7 for ICFs, and 29.2 for those not certified.[4] The ratios also vary by ownership. The proprietaries have the lowest ratio; the voluntaries, the highest. However, the overall average is rising. Staffing remains an almost universal problem. Registered nurses are hard to recruit. Sixty-six percent of all nursing home personnel are aides, generally working at minimum wage levels. Turnover is very high. Geriatric training is minimal and physician involvement sparse.

The nursing home industry today represents an interesting but still unstable compromise between the Medicare emphasis on short-term posthospital recuperation and rehabilitation—a medical institution designed to run like a small hospital—and the Medicaid emphasis on low-cost "custodial" LTC. In this confusing environment it is perhaps surprising that there has been any progress. Despite the documented persistence of poor quality and other serious abuses,[10–12] as well as a great deal of well-intentioned but mediocre care, there is no question but that the average home has improved dramatically since 1965. Whether this improvement will continue or whether a new phase of deterioration will set in, triggered by the recent cutbacks in Medicaid and Medicare and the Reagan Administration's apparent commitment to reduced regulation, remains to be seen. Again, in the words of the General Accounting Office,[12a]

Survey data indicate that patients entering nursing homes over the past several years are increasingly dependent or disabled; this trend is likely to continue. A more disabled nursing home population may imply a need for more extensive, and potentially more costly, care.

At the same time, States are finding it difficult to pay the escalating cost of this care and are taking steps to reduce their nursing home expenditures. . . . States are cutting reimbursement rates, freezing bed supply, and taking other actions that may change both the quality of nursing home care and patients' access to it.

Because these conflicting trends—increased patient needs for care versus State efforts to cut the cost of that care—are likely to continue over the next several years, the type of care provided to Medicaid patients is likely to change significantly.

Ironically, the effort to hold down nursing home costs by restricting bed supply may have contributed to even greater public costs. A 1980 study by the Office of the Inspector General for the Secretary of Health and Human Services reports that "backed up" patients, awaiting nursing home placement, average 10 percent of hospital occupancy. Medicare paid the bill for two-thirds of these patients[13]—the primary cause of the estimated $1.6 billion that Medicare paid for LTC in hospitals in 1980 (Table 1).

There is also no question that, compared to hospitals, hotels, or other institutions, the nursing home still provides a relatively cheap form of care. In 1977, the average monthly charge was $689, varying from a low of $670 in the proprietary homes to a high of $747 in the voluntaries (Table 2A). In terms of certification, the average charge varied from $880 for a SNF down to $390 for those not certified. Needless to say, rates have gone up a great deal since 1977—according to the U.S. Bureau of Labor Statistics by approximately the same amount as the hospital component of the consumer price index—roughly 14 percent.[14] This would bring the current average to something over $1,500 per month.

The enormous sums spent on nursing homes today reflect the growing population at risk, the increasing severity of disability among residents,[12a] the lengthy average stays, the rising personnel/bed ratios, and other qualitative improvements, rather than any large-scale exploitation or unconscionable profits. To the extent that qualitative improvement continues, e.g., through greater physician involvement[15] and the development of "teaching nursing homes" as recommended by leading geriatricians,[16] per diem costs will inevitably rise even more. According to the Health Care Financing Administration, (HCFA), total expenditures are expected to reach $67 billion by 1990.[6] Current approaches to regulation and reimbursement are frequently criticized,[4,11,17,18] but appropriate alternatives will not be easy to achieve.

Community-based Programs

The community-based segment of the LTC industry comprises a heterogeneous collection of agencies, institutions, and programs, public and private, whose chief common denominator is a commitment to noninstitutional health and health-related social services to the chronically ill and disabled, especially the elderly. According to the estimates in Table 1, this group accounted for $6.5 billion in 1980, 20 percent of all LTC expenditures in that year. Since there is no agreed-on definition as to its boundaries, such an estimate is inevitably arbitrary. However, it does help to indicate the order of magnitude and importance of this rapidly growing segment of the health care economy.

The listing and classification in Table 3, which are much broader than the items included in Table 1, are based primarily on material developed in HCFA's Office of Policy Analysis in 1980.[19] No such listing will prove universally acceptable. For example, the boundaries between health-related housing and general housing for the elderly are almost impossible to identify. In New Jersey, where nursing home beds have been strictly controlled and less than 4 percent of the elderly are in nursing homes (as compared to a national average of 5 percent), the number of elderly in boarding or "residential health care" facilities now exceeds the number in nursing home beds. It is very hard to distinguish between the characteristics of these two sets of patients. Vladeck has pointed out "the interconnectedness between long-term care needs and services on the one hand, and income support, housing, and social support for the frail elderly on the other . . . frail old people have to live somewhere, and well-managed congregate or supported housing can substitute for institutionalization."[20] One institution which addresses this "interconnectedness" very effectively for those who can afford it is the life care or continuing care retirement community.[21,21a]

Another question: should hospice care be included or not? It is omitted here, although there are persuasive arguments both pro and con. If time permitted, I think I would include it.

Even with the HCFA classifications, it is impossible to obtain consistent data showing longitudinal changes and developments. Although there is general agreement as to the dramatic growth and proliferation that has taken place, especially during the 1970s, the initial numbers were so small and the provider institutions

TABLE 3   Community-Based Long-Term Care Programs

Protected living arrangements
  Personal/domiciliary care facilities
    Personal care facilities usually provide assistance with three or more activities of daily living, e.g., bathing, eating, toileting, transferring, ambulation; domiciliary facilities, only one or two. Must be licensed in most states. No Medicare or Medicaid reimbursements but residents generally pay with Supplemental Security Income, supplemented by some states.
  Foster homes
    Private homes providing meals, housekeeping, minimum surveillance, and personal care. States may use Social Security Act Title XX money for this purpose.
  Congregate housing/retirement communities
    Age-separated housing for the elderly, providing on-site meals and minimum surveillance. Assistance for construction available from the Department of Housing and Human Development.
  Life care (continuing care) retirement communities
    A special category of housing and retirement community which also provides lifetime nursing home care if needed. Privately funded. Fairly expensive; generally considered beyond means of most elders but may be ideal for several millions of upper- and middle-class individuals or couples.
Home care
  Home health care
    Includes skilled nursing, physical, occupational, and speech therapy, medical social services, home health aide assistance, and medical supplies and appliances. Generally provided or supervised by Visiting Nurse Association personnel. Medicare reimbursement limited to the "homebound" and those in need of skilled nursing care, i.e., generally post-hospital recuperation. Medicaid less restrictive in terms of physical condition but highly restrictive in terms of income eligibility. All Medicare/Medicaid services formally under physician supervision.
  Personal care/homemaker/chore services
    Assistance with activities of daily living intended to keep elderly at home and avoid institutionalization. Limited reimbursement under Medicaid and Social Security Act titles III and XX.
  Home delivery/congregate meals
    "Meals on wheels" or meals provided in communal locations, e.g., churches and senior citizen centers. Funding primarily private; some from titles III and XX.
Adult day care
  Community-based programs intended to help isolated individuals remain at home. Vary widely although most provide lunch, social activities, dietary counseling, and instruction in personal hygiene. Limited Medicaid and titles III and XX funding.

SOURCE: Adapted from Department of Health and Human Services, Health Care Financing Administration. Long-Term Care: Background and Future Directions. Washington, D.C.: 1981.

so disparate that consistent information does not exist. For example, in the National Health Accounts, updated annually by the Division of National Cost Estimates in HCFA, there is no separate category for any of these community-based programs. Even the home health agencies have no separate identity in these accounts. A note explains that "estimates for home health agencies that are not hospital-based are added to the private income of other unspecified health professionals."[7] One would probably have to go back 40 to 50 years in the history of acute care health accounting in the United States to find such a dearth of essential information.

The balance of this section is limited to a discussion of home health care, where at least some fragmentary data are available. For example, it has been estimated that there are now some 5,700 home health agencies or programs in the United States; some 3,800 of these are certified for Medicare–Medicaid coverage.[22]

The contemporary home health agency is a fascinating hybrid with roots going back to various origins.[23] Most important perhaps is the legacy of public health nursing which emerged in the mid-1800s. Hospital-based programs can be traced back to 1796, when the Boston Dispensary established a home care program primarily as a way to train resident physicians. However, a century and a half passed before the next major hospital-based experiments, this time by Montefiore and St. Vincent's hospitals in New York City.[24,25] Even then, there was little emulation until the current hospital financial crunch made all types of outpatient care appear more attractive. For several decades, home nursing care was offered by life insurance companies. The comprehensive home care model, developed in Britain after World War II under the National Health Service, attracted and influenced some American planners, geriatricians, and gerontologists. Beginning in the 1950s, home nursing agencies began to augment their services with home health aides/homemakers, a new and still controversial paraprofessional category at least partially legitimized by Medicare and Medicaid.

Finally, an entirely new ingredient has been added—the technologically oriented, for-profit home health enterprise—a development encouraged by the 1980 removal of Medicare's former ban on reimbursement of for-profit home health services. Perhaps the best known example is the home dialysis business.[26] A complete newcomer is Home Health Care of America, a California-based national organization that specializes in parenteral feeding of posthospitalization patients at home and that reportedly increased its revenues from $1 million in 1981 to $40 million in 1982.[27] A consulting firm has projected a $16 billion market for this type of home care by 1990.

This rich, varied, and diffuse genealogy is reflected in the wide variety of home health agency sponsorship today. Table 4 shows the distribution by ownership in 1977 and 1981. Although government still accounts for 40 percent nationwide, its share is falling, as is that of the Visiting Nurse Association, while the three categories—hospital-based, proprietary, and private nonprofit—are growing. Even more dramatic is the tremendous regional variation: while government agencies accounted for 65 percent of the total in the West North Central states in 1981, they represented only 15 percent in the Pacific states. The proprietaries, nonexistent in New England, accounted for 23 percent in the Pacific region. Clearly, home health agencies and their personnel march to different drummers in different parts of the country.[28]

One measure of the rapid expansion in home health services derives from Medicare and Medicaid data (Table 5). These services increased under both programs but most dramatically under Medicaid, with a 20 percent average annual rate of growth in recipients (1973–1979) and nearly 40 percent in payments. The significance of these figures is considerably lessened when one realizes that, even in 1980, home health expenditures amounted to only 1.4 percent of all Medicaid expenditures and 2 percent of Medicare expenditures; also, that 77 percent of all Medicaid home health payments went to one state, New York.[29,30] Nevertheless, it is indicative of both the demand and the industry's ability to respond to that demand, given even modest fi-

TABLE 4 Home Health Agencies, Percentage Distribution by Type of Agency, 1977 and 1981

Type	1977	1981
Visiting Nurse Assn.	19	17
Government	47	40
Hospital-based	11	14
Proprietary	5	8
Private nonprofit	14	18
Other	4	3
Total	100	100

SOURCE: Home Health Line, Vol. VI, February 26, 1982, p. 2. Data from Health Care Financing Administration.

TABLE 5 Home Health Services, Use, and Reimbursement Under Medicare and Medicaid, Selected Years, 1970–1980

Year	Medicare		Medicaid	
	Visits (1,000s)	Reimbursements (millions)	Recipients (1,000s)	Payments (millions)
1970	6,000	$61.5	109.9[a]	25.4[a]
1975	10,900	217.0	202.4	70.3
1977	15,600	366.5	363.1	180.0
1979	19,200	518.2	358.4	262.6
1980	22,400	662.1	—	—
ACRG (%)[b]	9.2	21.4	19.7	39.0

[a]1973.

[b]ACRG, annual compound rate of growth. Medicare: 1969–1980; Medicaid: 1973–1979.

SOURCE: Muse, D.N., and Sawyer, D. Medicare and Medicaid Data Book, 1981. Baltimore, Md.: Health Care Financing Administration Publication No. 03128, 1982.

nancial incentives. The rate of growth under Medicaid should be even greater since 1981, when federal legislation provided for waivers to permit state coverage of home- and community-based services to recipients who would otherwise require institutional placement, provided such benefits do not exceed the cost of institutionalization (Omnibus Budget Reconciliation Act of 1981, Sec. 2176). Medicare waivers are also available under a limited number of demonstration projects (see below).

Long-Term Hospitals

Data on this segment of the industry, often omitted from discussion of LTC, are shown in Table 6, based on American Hospital Association classifications and data. Despite substantial shrinkage in the number of such institutions, over the past decade, especially in the number of beds, this group of hospitals still represents a substantial national resource. As of 1981, it accounted for 563 institutions, over 250,000 beds, 550,000 admissions, and expenditures over $8 billion.

Whether these hospitals will continue to shrink in number and size depends on many factors, including the adequacy of mainstream health care financing, the strength of the continuing shift

TABLE 6 Long-Term Hospitals,[a] United States, Selected Indicators, 1981

Classification	Hospitals	Beds	Admissions	Average Daily Census	Occupancy Rate (%)	Full-time Equivalent Personnel	Total Expenses (1,000s)
Psychiatric	394	205,003	423,867	177,742	85.3	274,588	$6,420,745
Federal	22	19,051	65,185	16,713	87.7	27,569	770,740
State	251	170,076	293,857	147,655	86.8	218,475	4,823,475
Local	4	2,098	2,026	1,750	83.4	2,422	69,286
Private nonprofit	52	6,944	26,886	6,153	88.6	14,162	383,998
Investor-owned	65	6,834	35,913	5,471	80.1	11,960	373,246
Tuberculosis and other respiratory diseases	10	1,492	7,626	1,000	65.8	2,744	62,122
State	8	1,299	6,752	876	67.4	2,191	49,346
Local	1	94	478	86	91.5	298	4,191
Private nonprofit	1	99	396	38	38.4	255	8,585
All other[b]	159	44,397	117,825	38,311	81.7	73,115	1,667,317
Federal	13	9,180	40,884	7,960	76.3	12,491	358,969
State	37	12,030	18,314	9,969	72.7	15,991	339,986
Local	30	11,451	17,203	10,210	85.7	20,110	390,859
Private nonprofit	69	10,474	34,870	9,067	86.1	21,836	515,628
Investor-owned	10	1,259	6,554	1,105	87.8	2,687	71,875
Total	563	250,892	549,318	217,053	86.5	350,447	$8,160,184

[a]Average length-of-stay is 30 days or more.
[b]Includes institutions for the mentally retarded, alcoholism and other chemical dependencies, other chronic diseases, rehabilitation, etc.

SOURCE: American Hospital Association. Hospital Statistics, 1982 Ed., Chicago, pp. 10–11.

to community programs, the degree of flexibility permitted the hospitals with respect to level of care, the state of the general economy, and of course financial incentives from the major financing programs. Of special interest is the transfer of hundreds of thousands of former psychiatric patients to nursing homes, i.e., a transfer from state to at least partial federal support that is a striking example of the impact of different financial arrangements and incentives on the utilization and size of different types of institutions that in no way reduces the overall costs of care. For example, expenditures for long-term psychiatric hospitals rose from $3.4 billion in 1971[31] to $6.4 billion in 1981 (Table 6). For all long-term hospitals, the rise was from $4.7 billion to $8.2 billion.

Summarizing, it is clear that there is now in place an extensive and expensive LTC industry, however defined. Despite these substantial resources, the current product of our LTC industry falls far short of the suggested goal—maximum functional independence of the elderly and disabled. On the contrary, there has been no significant reduction in the proportion of elderly who are institutionalized or disabled.*[32] Responsibility for the shortfall does not necessarily rest with the industry itself. Some blame the financing programs and incentives to which the industry has responded, in short, public policy—or the lack of it.

II. PAYING FOR LONG-TERM CARE

The proportion of LTC expenditures met through public funds, 61 percent (Table 1), is much higher than that for the nation's overall health care bill, 43 percent,[7] but is about the same as for all personal health care expenditures for the elderly, 63 percent.[8] Within the public sphere, however, there is considerable difference between federal and state/local participation in LTC compared to all health care. Whereas state and local governments paid for only 13 percent of all expenditures, they paid 19 percent for LTC. One big difference, of course, is the federal Medicare program, which accounts for over 40 percent of all health care

---

*It should be kept in mind that the majority of elderly were not, and are not, disabled. According to the National Center for Health Statistics, over two-thirds of all noninstitutionalized elderly perceived their own health as "excellent" or "good" in 1980. An estimated 55 percent had no limitation of activity. (Ref. 9.)

expenditures for the elderly but a very small portion of LTC expenditures. The Medicare estimates in Table 1, which come to 9 percent of total LTC expenditures, are probably exaggerated by some definitional anomalies.

Within the private sphere there is also a dramatic difference. Whereas private health insurance accounts for over one-fourth of total health care expenditures, its contribution to the financing of LTC is very small. Again, the figures in Table 1 are probably high. Nearly one-third of all LTC expenditures are still paid out-of-pocket by consumers.

Following is a summary of the major LTC financing programs. We start with Medicare only because it is synonymous with U.S. health policy for the elderly. It is impossible to understand or even to discuss such policy intelligently without recognizing the void that Medicare created by failure to cover LTC, a void that other programs have tried to fill without benefit of any public or professional leadership or guidance.

Medicare

Following the private health insurance pattern, dominant in the early 1960s, Medicare focuses almost exclusively on short-term acute care. Section 1862 of the law specifically prohibits payment for "custodial" care and the meaning of "custodial" is spelled out in the official *Medicare Handbook* as follows:

Care is considered custodial when it is primarily for the purpose of meeting personal needs and could be provided by persons without professional skills or training. For example, custodial care includes help in walking, getting in and out of bed, bathing, dressing, eating, and taking medicine.

Obviously, these skills, which Medicare dismisses so contemptuously, are precisely those needed by the long-term stroke patient, the patient with Alzheimer's or Parkinson's disease, multiple sclerosis, terminal cancer, or any number of other chronic conditions. The tragic irony, of course, is that Medicare will, and does, pay generously for the same patient after he or she has developed an infected bedsore, or a circulatory blockage, or pneumonia, from failure to get out of bed or ambulate to whatever limits are possible. This is justified as a separate "episode of illness"—a concept that is increasingly obsolete in a context of chronic disease.

Not only does Medicare prohibit reimbursement for nursing home care beyond 100 days, but this is available only following hospitalization, only in a SNF, and only when the patient is in need of skilled nursing care, which is arbitrarily and inconsistently interpreted by both the administrative intermediaries and the Department of Health and Human Services.[33] More and more it appears that the difference between "custodial care" and "skilled nursing care" has little to do with the degree of skill required, but a great deal to do with the patient's prognosis. The Medicare message to the seriously ill patient is clear, "get well fast, die, or get lost—unless you can qualify for another acute 'episode' "!

Spokesmen for Medicare are defensive on this point. They point out that the program is a godsend not only to elderly patients experiencing a first stroke or heart attack, but whenever there is an acute exacerbation of a chronic condition. That is correct. But what distinguishes chronic disease from most acute disease and trauma is not the absence of such acute episodes but the usually slow and insidious onset and the frequently lengthy period of disability. The latter may, or may not, be interrupted by acute episodes but, no matter how well such episodes are handled medically, by definition the condition is never "cured." If the goal of LTC is maximum functional independence for the chronically disabled patient, then the incentives to the system and to individual professionals should be continued improvement, rehabilitation, and the prevention of acute episodes—not just meeting them when the need arises, in at least some cases precisely because continuing care was denied.

Only in the field of home health services has Medicare demonstrated some sensitivity to the growing needs of the chronically ill and the importance of linkage between acute care and LTC. From the beginning, both the hospitalization (Part A) and physician service (Part B) coverage authorized up to 100 home health visits per year by a part-time skilled nurse or therapist, under physician certification and supervision. Also, in a departure from private health insurance norms, Medicare permitted use of a home health aide—if one of the skilled professionals was also needed. However, to emphasize the short-term nature of the benefit, Part A required at least a three-day prior hospitalization. Then, starting in 1981, the home health benefit was liberalized, at least on paper. The Part A prior hospitalization requirement was eliminated and the 100-visit limit removed, although the limitations inherent in the requirement for skilled nursing remain. As noted, for-profit home health agencies are now permitted to qualify.

At the present writing, it is too soon to evaluate the impact of the new home health amendments. Home health personnel claim that regulations have been tightened to the point where the statutory liberalization has been more than cancelled out. In fact, the use of home health aides has been further restricted from a maximum of 20 to 9 hours per week. At least in concept, however, Medicare has now gone beyond its private health insurance model in recognizing the need for long-term home health services.

Despite failure to cover LTC as well as preventive services, which many feel could help to prevent or postpone the incidence of a great deal of chronic illness and disability, and despite sporadic Reagan Administration efforts at cost control, Medicare reimbursement soared at an average annual rate of over 17 percent to $36 billion in 1980,[29,30] an estimated $57 billion in fiscal year 1983 and a projected $76 billion for 1985. In one fiscal year, 1980–1981, the rise was 21 percent. The Hospital Insurance (Part A) Trust Fund is expected to be bankrupt before the end of the decade.[34] In an effort to stem the rise, drastic changes in the program are now being effected and more are proposed.[35,36]

Private Health Insurance

Although private health insurance in the United States preceded Medicare by over three decades and greatly influenced the philosophy and benefit structure of the public program, once Medicare became law, the two programs were neatly fitted together in a mutually complementary relationship. The basic definition of covered benefits in most private insurance policies, including major medical policies, is the same as in Medicare. Both share the same acute, inpatient bias.

The widely held "Medicare supplementary" or "Medigap" policies, sold both by Blue Cross–Blue Shield and the insurance companies, are intended primarily to fill the gaps resulting from Medicare deductibles and co-insurance and an occasional uncovered benefit such as private duty nursing. The Medigap experience is significant in demonstrating the widespread public craving for comprehensive coverage and the difficulty of relying on patient cost-sharing as an effective method of cost control. As presently conceived and marketed, however, private insurance is simply not a significant factor in the financing of LTC for the elderly. In 1981, for example, it paid for 0.2 percent of nursing home expenses.[7]

The new Medicare requirement that private insurance, rather than Medicare, must be the first payor of benefits to patients over 65 who are still working will create many new difficulties for older workers and their insurers, but will have little or no effect on LTC.

Medicaid

Along with direct patient or family payment, Medicaid is the primary source of funding for LTC in the United States, especially nursing home care. As of 1980, some 1.8 million individuals, over 8 percent of all Medicaid recipients, were receiving one of the three principal long-term services—in a skilled nursing facility, intermediate care facility, or home health care—and this does not include the mentally retarded or those receiving only prescribed drugs.[30] As to costs, Medicaid made 1980 vendor payments of over $8 billion for these three services, over 35 percent of total payments that year. At the same time, LTC providers, especially institutional providers, received a shot-in-the-arm from the substantial infusion of new Medicaid money. In 1981, Medicaid paid 56 percent of all U. S. nursing home expenditures. Some authorities maintain that the American nursing home is largely a creation of Medicaid and its predecessor, Kerr–Mills Medical Assistance for the Aged.

However, this is clearly a hen-and-egg relationship. Just as the nursing home has been molded by Medicaid's welfare orientation, Medicaid itself has been vastly changed by the impact of its most expensive provider. In fact, it is now widely acknowledged that Medicaid is not one but two or even three programs, depending on the category of recipient. Those 65 and over constitute only 16 percent of total recipients but account for 37 percent of the cost.[29]

Although poor, nearly 40 percent of these elderly are *not* on welfare and this 40 percent accounts for nearly three-quarters of all Medicaid expenditures for this age group. This is primarily the nursing home population—formerly self-supporting individuals forced to "spend down" to the level of penury that qualifies them for a Medicaid nursing home bed. Add the under-65 disabled and the total is still less than 30 percent of recipients but accounts for over 67 percent of all payments. By contrast, families receiving funds from Aid to Families with Dependent Children programs, the stereotypical "welfare patients," account for almost two-thirds of all recipients but less than 30 percent of payments. However unintended or unplanned was Medicaid's move into the long-term field, it did so, to the credit of its administrators at both federal and state levels.

Despite Medicaid's contribution to LTC, however, many deep-seated problems remain. Most obvious is the fact that the program covers only the very poor—in 1980 about 3.5 million out of a total of 25.7 million over 65, approximately 13 percent.[30,37] (The actual number of recipients was 3.4 million but the HCFA estimates another 100,000 or so who were eligible did not participate in 1980). In New Jersey, the figure is only 5 to 6 percent. Closely related is the inconsistency in eligibility and benefit provisions among the 54 jurisdictions. For example, 20 states limit eligibility to those on Supplementary Security Income. Of those that do cover the "medically needy," income limits vary as much as 3:1.

Second, there is the persistent problem of political and financial instability inherent in a "welfare" program. Despite recent reported progress in some states in restraining costs, Medicaid remains the fastest growing financial burden for many and the LTC segment the fastest growing part of that burden. Already freed of many of the original federal requirements relating to such matters as mandatory benefits, provider payment, and patients' exercise of free choice, and faced with the federal cuts decreed in 1981, the states feel forced to cut and pinch still further. This creates hardship not only for recipients but for the providers, e.g., responsible nursing home operators or home health agencies who find advance planning and quality maintenance extremely difficult, if not impossible.

It is not surprising that a large proportion of providers, especially the better ones, refuse Medicaid patients altogether. For example, there is wide variation in the number and proportion of participating physicians in the different states. An incomplete 1982 survey reported that the ratio of participating physicians per 1,000 Medicaid recipients ranged from 7.13 in Pennsylvania to 39.39 in Wyoming.[38]

An earlier study, using 1976 data, found that nearly 60 percent of all Medicaid patients treated in private practices were seen in less than 15 percent of all such practices.[39] While the authors of this study rejected all allegations that most of these large Medicaid practices were "Medicaid mills" in the sense of flagrantly abusing or exploiting the system, they did find a substantial "credentials gap." "The Medicaid market," they wrote, "is dominated by less qualified physicians . . . older, non-board certified, and graduates of foreign medical schools."

Third, there is the basic incompatibility between Medicaid and the goal of a good LTC program as set forth at the beginning of this paper. Continuity of care is almost impossible as the elderly patient's care is fragmented between Medicare and Medicaid or whatever other source of assistance for LTC may be available to the 87 percent who do not qualify for Medicaid, as well as between medical and social services. This fragmentation will probably increase with the current push toward alternative sources of care, and even those fortunate elders who still have family doctors may be forced to leave them in favor of some health care corporation with which the state has signed a contract. Also, care remains generally biased in favor of the most expensive modality, i.e., institutional care.

The positive aspects of the 1981 provisions for waivers to permit states to provide expanded home- and community-based services to Medicaid patients who would otherwise require nursing home placement may be cancelled out by the negative implications of other waivers permitting denial of free choice to Medicaid patients.

Perhaps most important of all is the basic conflict imposed on patient and family incentives between a welfare program and the goal of good LTC—maximum functional independence. By limiting eligibility to those already seriously dependent, both medically and financially, or to those who make themselves dependent for this purpose (now called "targeting to the at-risk population"), the program not only fails to encourage independent functioning but actually promotes dependency of both types. In a 1974 survey, the Congressional Budget Office found that nearly half of Medicaid nursing home patients were not initially poor by state definitions but were forced to deplete their resources in order to qualify as "medically needy."[40] This percentage has almost certainly increased since that time.

A 1980 study by the former Assistant Commissioner of Health of New Jersey[41] notes that:

Children are not financially responsible for the care of parents . . . but spouses are; hence the phenomenon of couples married 50 years divorcing to enable one of them to get nursing home subsidy without totally impoverishing the other.

The spend-down for nursing home care presents many middle-class families with an excruciating dilemma. Either they violate the law by covertly attempting to transfer the parent's assets before admission to the nursing home . . . or they can watch passively an inheritance go up in smoke. For those families unable or unwilling to transfer assets covertly, nursing home services have thus become the most effective barrier to intergenerational transfer of income ever seen in this country.

This orientation may be inevitable in a relatively small, residual, "salvage" type of program, such as Medicaid was originally intended to be. However, as the program has expanded to cover hundreds of thousands of formerly hardworking, middle-class patients, such an orientation becomes increasingly inappropriate.

Despite all these supposedly cost-saving limits and many more, the costs of Medicaid increased, at least through 1979, at an average annual rate of 13.6 percent.[29] Since 1981, the rate of increase has declined considerably, to an estimated 10 percent in 1982–1983.[36] Nevertheless, total vendor payments—$23 billion in 1980[30]—are projected to reach $39 billion in 1984. No wonder many states are grappling with a very difficult dilemma: how to cut the costs of Medicaid while assuring that basic medical services are available to the poor.[42]

Title XX

Title XX of the Social Security Act (1974) provides federal block grants to the states for a broad range of social services to poor people all ages, based on eligibility standards determined, since 1981, by the states. It has become "the major source of funding for noncash benefit social service for a broad array of client groups ranging from female-headed single-parent, poor families to mentally retarded children, to working poor families, to pregnant teenagers, to the elderly."[42a] In this broad pool of social problems, the elderly are by no means predominant. It is estimated that 6 to 10 percent of total funds go to them. While the emphasis remains on the poor, the greater state administrative latitude since 1981 has resulted in opening up Title XX funds to nonpoor groups such as the nonpoor elderly.

The states also have wide latitude in defining services. Those of particular interest to the elderly include day care and senior centers, homemakers, home health aides, personal care, consumer education, and financial counseling. Institutional care is excluded.

In 1980, an estimated $809 million were spent on LTC services under Title XX (Table 1), about 30 percent of a total appropriation of $2.5 billion. Three years later, in 1983, the total was $2.45 billion,[43] a fairly significant cut considering inflation. Such retrenchment, coupled with wide state latitude in setting group priorities, has led to growing intrastate competition for the available funds.

A separate Community Services Block Grant program provides many of the same services as Title XX but is generally targeted to minority groups and administered through separate local agencies. Appropriations for this program in 1983 were $361 million.[43]

Older Americans Act

The Older Americans Act of 1965 and its subsequent amendments created a national/state/local service network for the elderly, generally defined as those 60 +. (States have considerable latitude in establishing eligibility criteria for services other than nutrition.) The Administration on Aging was set up within the Department of Health and Human Services and federal money was allotted to states that paid their smaller share—75/25 for administration, 85/15 for services—and through them to some 700 area agencies on aging. The latter enjoy a high degree of autonomy. Means testing is prohibited, permitting this program to reach those elderly who are ineligible for Medicaid or Title XX.

Community health services funded through this Act include, under Title III, visiting nurses, homemaker/home health aides, health education, screening and immunization, home-delivered meals, other nutrition programs, and home repairs; and under Title IV, research and demonstration projects to develop alternatives to institutionalization and improve service delivery, education, etc. Expenditures for 1980 came to $724 million (Table 1); in 1983, to $954 million, a slight increase over 1982. (1982–1983 figures may not be strictly comparable to 1980).[43]

Veterans Administration Programs

The Veterans Administration (VA) operates the largest medical service in the United States, with some 400 facilities and 200,000 doctors, nurses, and other employees, treating about 1.3 million patients a year at a current cost of nearly $8 billion.[44] One hundred and seventy-two acute care hospitals represent the traditional core of the VA Medical Center system. Recognizing the rapid aging of the veteran population, however, the VA has embarked on an ambitious new geriatric program, involving both the expansion of existing facilities and services and the deliberate reorientation of existing resources toward LTC. Among the new developments:

• The number of beds in long-term or extended care facilities is being increased.

• Eight Geriatric Research, Educational, and Clinical centers have been established in VA medical centers around the country for research into aging and geriatric care and for the education of health professionals in such care.

• Five adult health care centers are operating as demonstration projects to explore outpatient treatment of the elderly.

• A variety of programs have been established in community, state, and VA homes to care for patients with chronic conditions.

• A palliative treatment center has been established in Los Angeles to study the latest developments in the care of the terminally ill.

• A geriatric fellowship program has been established for physicians; now in its fifth year, its largest class graduated in 1983.

In terms of dollars and other resources, the new LTC programs are still overshadowed by acute care (total VA expenditures in 1980 for LTC are estimated at $2.6 billion; see Table 1), as in the general U.S. health care economy. But there is a significant difference. The VA leadership appears to understand the "geriatric imperative" and is committed to trying to meet it as effectively and humanely as possible, even if this involves some transfers of resources. A significant portion of VA research is also targeted to this end.

In the words of the agency director, H. N. Walters, "The VA is on the cutting edge of the problem of a graying America."[45] And Dr. J. H. Mather, Assistant Chief Medical Director for Geriatric and Extended Care, said recently, "There is a feeling that we're breaking ground on one of the most important problems facing the country. It's exciting stuff."

In the effort to strengthen the new thrust, a Special Medical Advisory Group Task Force on the Geriatric Plan was convened in the spring of 1983. Its report[46] begins with the following statement of objective:

The maintenance and restoration of optimal patient functioning is critical to the care of the aged patient . . . The central objective of care is the maintenance or improvement of functioning . . . accomplished through prevention, the delivery of appropriate health services, and rehabilitation.

Other points were emphasized in the report:

• There is a need for a continuum of care, ranging from home and community-based services to institutional care.

• Because of the varied, complex array of health-related interventions required, geriatric services must be coordinated, both between disciplines and across levels of care. Coordination is characterized by multidisciplinary patient assessment, case management, tracking and monitoring, and follow-up. The VA must identify and remove impediments to patient flow, across levels of care, among patient care services, and between VA and non-VA providers.

Needless to say, such statements assume special significance in a setting where policy directives can be translated directly into operating programs. The potential of the VA geriatric experiments also becomes clearer when one realizes that by the year 2000, two out of every three men over 65 and one out of three in the entire elderly population will be veterans. Moreover, since 1970 all veterans have been automatically eligible for health care, regardless of disability or of financial status. Today only 15 to 25 percent of older veterans use VA services. But this could change dramatically if other sources fail to provide the financial support for needed LTC. The financial incentives involved are not obscure.

The incredible mish-mash of overlapping federal programs providing some type of LTC to the chronically impaired elderly is

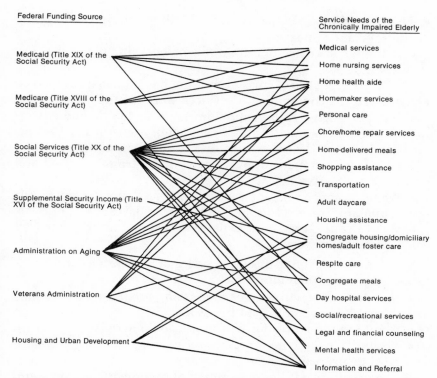

Federal Funding Source

Service Needs of the
Chronically Impaired Elderly

Medicaid (Title XIX of the
Social Security Act)

Medicare (Title XVIII of the
Social Security Act)

Social Services (Title XX of the
Social Security Act)

Supplemental Security Income (Title
XVI of the Social Security Act)

Administration on Aging

Veterans Administration

Housing and Urban Development

Medical services

Home nursing services

Home health aide

Homemaker services

Personal care

Chore/home repair services

Home-delivered meals

Shopping assistance

Transportation

Adult daycare

Housing assistance

Congregate housing/domiciliary
homes/adult foster care

Respite care

Congregate meals

Day hospital services

Social/recreational services

Legal and financial counseling

Mental health services

Information and Referral

FIGURE 1 Major Federal Programs Funding Community Services for the Elderly. From U.S. General Accounting Office. Entering a Nursing Home—Costly Implications for Medicaid and the Elderly. Report to the Congress. Washington, D.C.: 1979, p. 74.

shown in Figure 1. If state/local, voluntary, and for-profit programs were added, the confusion would be compounded to the point of chaos. It is surprising that the "nonsystem" works as well as it does, but not surprising that the costs are so high.

Obviously, more than money is needed to straighten out this mess. The Reagan Administration is correct in that view. But, if not money, then what? The situation will not solve itself. And, if money is not to provide the carrot, what incentives are there to efficiency, quality, and more equitable access?

Community-Based LTC Demonstration Projects

The need for a more coordinated and efficient approach to LTC has been recognized for several years. The January 1981 Report of HCFA's Office of Policy Analysis[19] correctly identified many of the relevant issues:

- Is there a shortage of nursing home beds and if so, what are its consequences?
- What percentage of current nursing home residents could be cared for in the community if services were available?
- Can currently available preadmission screening and assessment mechanisms identify high risk populations in need of services and thus delay or prevent institutionalization?
- Can case management overcome system fragmentation and assure cost-effective use of LTC services?
- Would expanded noninstitutional services supplement rather than supplant present informal family/friends' care?
- What are the costs and benefits of expanding in-home and community-based services?

The report went on to discuss a series of five options and strategies for reform, including:

- incremental modifications of existing programs,
- comprehensive grants to the states,
- grants to the states for noninstitutional services,
- disability payments for LTC, and
- LTC insurance.

Space prohibits a fuller description of this report, but it should be considered an appendix to this paper. The change in administration and the growing federal budgetary difficulties precluded strong federal leadership along any of these lines. Aside from the VA programs, the major federal contribution to the growing LTC dilemma has been the continued funding of several series of demonstration projects, focused primarily on questions 2 to 6 cited above from the HCFA Report.[19]

First were the 15 Medicaid/Medicare community-based LTC "waiver" projects;* second, the National LTC Channeling Demonstration Project with 10 sites.† A number of other programs

---

*These 15 projects are known by their names or locations, as follows: ACCESS, ACCESS II, Florida, Georgia, Mount Zion, Multi-Purpose Senior Services Project, New York City, New York State, On Lok, Oregon, San Diego, South Carolina, Texas, Triage, Wisconsin.

†The 10 sites are Miami, Florida; counties in eastern Kentucky; Baltimore, Maryland; Greater Lynn, Massachusetts; counties in southern Maine; Middlesex County, New Jersey; Rensselaer County, New York; Cuyahoga County (Cleveland), Ohio; Philadelphia, Pennsylvania; and Houston, Texas.

have been initiated by states and foundations. Results from the "waivers" projects are discussed in a 1982 report by the federal General Accounting Office.[47] It concluded that "expanded home health care can reduce nursing home use only for some subpopulations of the elderly; the effect of expanded home health care on hospital use is still unclear; some client outcome measures have shown improvement; while individual nursing home or hospital costs may have been reduced, total health care costs increased; methodological problems hamper the existing research results." To meet the GAO criticism, a second research effort is underway to combine comparable data from the sites. The new cross-cutting evaluation is focusing on eligibility, costs, client outcomes, service mix, remibursement, and financing mechanisms. Results are expected to be available in late 1983.

The "channeling" project represents the most rigorous LTC research effort to date. It focuses on community-based services for frail elders who would otherwise be eligible for institutionalization. Each site has an experimental and control group. Two models are being evaluated. Both include case management within the existing service system. Case management services include outreach and screening, assessment, care planning, arranging for services, monitoring, and reassessment. The five "basic" model sites offer limited funds to fill service gaps while the five "complex" sites may provide and authorize expanded service coverage through waivers, practice cost sharing, and utilize a funding pool. Resources are capped at 60 percent of nursing home costs. Preliminary results are schedule for release in March of 1984.[48]

Other experiments include HCFA's Social Health Maintenance Organization project, managed by Brandeis University and currently being implemented at four sites[49]; the New York State Long-Term Home Health Care Program, known as the Nursing Home Without Walls program; the Robert Wood Johnson Foundation project for the Health-Impaired Elderly; and the Hartford Foundation–Rutgers Medical School Geriatrics Demonstration Project, which explicitly focuses on health maintenance for young elders.[50] In a related experiment, the Oregon Region Kaiser-Permanente Medical Care Program has reported success with one of HCFA's Medicare Prospective Payment Demonstrations[51]; however, this did not involve LTC patients. The General Accounting Office report concludes, "The critical policy issue may not be whether one service is less costly than another but, rather, how new services should be organized to insure maximum efficiency and effectiveness."[47]

Packwood-Bradley-Heinz Bill

The major Congressional contribution to the growing LTC debate is S. 1244, the Senior Citizens Independent Community Care Act, introduced in May 1983. A bipartisan effort on the part of three leading senators from the Special Committee on Aging, S. 1244 would amend Title XVIII of the Social Security Act (Medicare) to authorize new state-administered capitation programs to include both acute care and LTC for the impaired elderly. During the first four years, only four states would qualify, but others could be added later as funds in the Part A Trust Fund permit.

In addition to the usual Medicare benefits, the program would provide homemaker/home health aide services (without existing Medicare restrictions), adult day services, up to 14 days of respite care and 20 days of ICF care per year, preadmission assessment, case management, and other services as authorized by the Secretary of Health and Human Services. To be eligible, an individual must be certified as "severely" or "moderately" impaired by a special preadmission assessment team. There would be a 20 percent co-payment on the costs of all services, with an annual limit varying with income.

The Secretary is instructed to report on the four initial programs at the end of four years, with recommendations for implementing the program nationally. Simultaneously, the Office of Management and Budget is to report on the budgetary impact.

Originally, this proposal was conceived solely as another demonstration project. The present version seeks to combine the demonstration aspect with the potential for national implementation. This could turn out to be a politically ingenious compromise—setting the stage for future national policy while holding down costs in the immediate future. However, another compromise, between the "medical model" and the "social model," is more problematic. Originally the authors had advanced the proposal as a new Title XXI program. At first glance, it would appear that the switch to Title XVIII brings the program closer to the Medicare mainstream. In fact, however, it might have the reverse effect. To obtain LTC benefits under the new program, Medicare beneficiaries would have to join special capitated plans set up for this purpose that control both LTC and acute care for their enrollees. Would the net effect be improved access and quality at least for those with frequent acute episodes? Obviously we are still far from the "last word," or even the "next to the last word," with respect to financing LTC in the United States.

III. INCENTIVES, ISSUES, AND RESEARCH SUGGESTIONS

Speaking to the American Medical Association on June 23, 1983, President Reagan said, "Our federal health care system was designed backwards. The incentives have not been to save, but to spend. Medicare and Medicaid costs have gone up nearly 600 percent since 1970."[52] The President was correct as to the incentives and the consequences. But the first sentence is meaningless. "Backwards" in relation to what? If President Johnson could be queried on the same issue, I suspect he would say that the Medicare/Medicaid incentives were fully compatible with the objectives of the Great Society health care programs, i.e., to open up access to hitherto underserved populations and to improve quality of care.

Today there is a widespread feeling, which I share,[53] that both objectives and incentives need to be modified and that cost constraints are essential. But beyond that generalization, there is very little agreement—virtually none in the LTC area. As Bruce Vladeck has pointed out, with respect to nursing homes, "It is hard to make a judgment on what the 'right' supply of institutional beds of any sort should be when there is no broad consensus about what these institutions should do."[54]

Moreover, we might as well be clear from the outset that a good LTC program for the elderly and disabled will never be cheap, any more than a good acute care program. On the contrary, every advance in acute care is likely to lead to additional cost in LTC—the "paradox of medical progress." In the United Kingdom, where the costs of all health care are tightly constrained, it has recently been reported that the treatment costs of the old now average nine times as much as the treatment of people of working age.[55] This is a startling statement since we in the United States tend to think in terms of 2.5:1 or 3:1.[9] Part of the difference may be the large amount of hidden LTC costs which, as already noted, are not now reflected in our National Health Accounts; part is undoubtedly unmet needs in this country.

Before rushing off to redesign the financing mechanisms of our LTC economy, or even to design large-scale research and development projects to test alternative mechanisms, it is essential first to come to some agreement on definitions, goals, and objectives. The following 12 points are suggested for consideration in developing a research agenda in LTC financing for the National Academy of Sciences—Institute of Medicine Committee on an Aging Society. The first three are very broad, value-laden, and difficult to study. But unless some degree of consensus is achieved in these areas, findings from the more specific, strictly financial, easier-to-get-at questions may turn out to be valueless, in a practical as well as philosophical sense.

In most cases the issues are presented as dichotomies, deliberately oversimplified in order to emphasize the existing polarity of views. Generally, I am convinced, appropriate public policy lies somewhere in the broad middle ground between these polarities. However, it is helpful to understand the extremes in order to arrive at a compromise.

1. *Basic Goal of Long-Term Care: Cure vs. Care?* This dichotomy is generally stated as "medical model vs. social model," a formulation which I find more provocative and less useful since it emphasizes the alleged turf battle between physicians and nonphysicians for control of the LTC field. Such a conflict may in fact be emerging, as noted in point 8 below. The issue, however, goes far beyond any such interprofessional competition and involves a basic difference in philosophy and objectives.

The arguments against the "cure" model for LTC are well known and persuasive: first, by definition, chronic disease is generally incurable. High-technology medicine is ill-suited to the long-term, often discouraging, demands of chronic illness, and the aversion of most physicians to nursing home and home care patients is undeniable. But can we, or should we, turn the clock back? Whether most providers like it or not, chronic disease is now the *central*, not a peripheral, challenge in modern health care. And the preservation or restoration of functional ability is, or should be, the central goal of such care,[56,57] not a secondary consideration to be delegated to nonphysicians when the physician has given up on the "interesting" aspects of a case, i.e., the diagnosis and treatment of reversible disease. The potential significance of this new approach was suggested recently by Dr. Robert Butler. Replying to a question as to whether we may be entering into a new era of hope for the elderly, he said,[58]

Definitely. We cannot prevent people from growing old and we cannot forestall death indefinitely. But we now have a chance to do something about the debilities of aging. We can intervene with treatments that relate to hormones, like estrogen; that relate to diet, such as calcium; and medications that control blood pressure, which is a high risk factor for strokes. And we have the new gerontology, which instead of focusing on disease, disability, and death, is beginning to get behind the underlying mechanisms of aging.

Indeed, most geriatricians think in terms of a *comprehensive* model that encompasses both curing (insofar as possible) and caring, the medical model and the social model, acute care and LTC. Among most third party payers, however, the dichotomy remains as rigid as the Iron Curtain. Is this accidental? Inevitable? Or a consequence of present methods of financing?

This paper started with a definition of LTC that seeks to combine the two goals. The large caring component is recognized in the long-term coverage, the need for a multidisciplinary approach, and some additional managerial functions. But the basic goals—maximum functional independence—preserves the activist, optimistic bias and related responsibilities characteristic of acute care medicine, as opposed to "custodial care."

Undoubtedly, the definition could be improved and the effort should be made, with inputs not only from all the relevant professions and interests in this country but from other countries with more, or different, experience. Such a definition of goal would then provide the baseline for evaluation of programs, agencies, and institutions seeking recognition in the LTC field, and for the design of appropriate financial incentives, including incentives for prevention and rehabilitation.

2. *Basic Eligibility for Long-Term Care: Medicare vs. Medicaid?* In sharp contrast to Medicare's near universal coverage of the elderly and seriously disabled, Medicaid eligibility involves a means test. Coverage is limited to the very poor—in most states only 5 to 10 percent of elderly. Aside from gross regional inequities, such discrimination against patients with long-term illness and disability is totally inconsistent with the central role

of chronic illness and disability in our society and the rapidly growing share of the national health dollar going to LTC, now on the order of $50 billion per year.

The effort to hold down costs and to husband resources for the acute care field is not only ethically untenable but is proving impractical as well. The question is not whether a greater proportion of the health care dollar will go to LTC or not. The questions are: How will this transfer be accomplished? How cost- and health-effective will the new arrangements prove to be? Will the majority of LTC patients benefit, or only a small, arbitrarily defined minority (e.g., New York State residents, who now consume about three-fourths of all Medicaid home health care funds)? Eligible veterans? Patients with end-stage renal disease? Can or should those special, favored categories be maintained in the future?

Elsewhere I have suggested that basic Medicare eligibility be extended to LTC benefits, the additional costs to be met by (1) transfer of Medicaid funds now used for LTC to Medicare; (2) fixed prices on all Medicare benefits, acute and LTC; and (3) reasonable cost-sharing for all patients.[59] Many disagree with this approach.[60] The costs and benefits of alternative proposals to provide financial protection to the growing legions of elderly LTC patients need prompt and careful study.

3. *Relation to Other Health Care Programs: Mainstream vs. Separate?* This issue overlaps with the two previous points. The case for a separate LTC system is often supported both by those who believe it to be very important and those who do not. The former stress their fear of the "medical model," especially as embodied in Medicare, and the inadequacies of high-technology medicine in relation to chronic illness and disability. At the same time, some supporters of the acute care system fear that extension of Medicare coverage to LTC could seriously dilute the funds now available for acute care.

Despite these understandable concerns and others that could be advanced, the case for programmatic integration, or at least close coordination, seems to me compelling. In the first place, even a well-funded LTC program, if separate from the acute care mainstream, will never achieve the same level of quality; it will remain a "stepchild," as Medicaid has been from the beginning. "Separate but equal" will not be equal in this area any more than in education. In the inevitable rationing of resources, it will be much easier to shortchange LTC if it is organizationally and financially separate from acute care.

Second, separation is not cost-effective. As already noted, despite the discrimination against LTC, the costs have grown astronomically. Nursing home and home care are now the fastest growing segments of the health care field. It may appear easier to limit Medicaid costs than those of Medicare but the final accounting has to consider the increased demands on the VA, uncompensated days in acute care hospitals, etc.

Moreover, one of the major causes of the current cost escalation is the duplication that inevitably results side by side with remaining gaps from a congeries of separate programs, such as shown in Figure 1. This is one of my chief worries in regard to S. 1244, the Packwood-Bradley-Heinz bill.

4. *Primary Financial Responsibility: Public vs. Private?*   Thus far, the private insurance industry has shown little interest in LTC, chiefly because the financial stakes seemed inconsequential and the potential market very poor.[61,62] The first of these conditions is changing, especially with the rapid growth in nursing home expenditures; and this could change the prospective market. There are some who now feel that new and "creative" financial instruments might enable private insurers to enter the market successfully.[63] Among these suggestions, probably the best known is the Social Health Maintenance Organization (S/HMO), already noted in Part II. Also mentioned is a possible Medical Retirement Account, modeled after the tax-subsidized Individual Retirement Account.[64] A three-pronged approach to community-based LTC has been suggested by James Firman of the Robert Wood Johnson Foundation,[65] including "home equity conversion options," "voluntary sector initiatives to provide home care for $1–5/hour," and "a voucher system for home care." Just how any of these would be tied in to the basic health care of the elderly is not clear.

My own feeling is that the carriers are well advised to be cautious. It was their inability to successfully underwrite acute care for the elderly and disabled that led to Medicare in the first place and I can see no reason to expect my better experience with LTC. There is, I feel sure, a significant role for private carriers and plans in the LTC field, but on a subsidiary basis.* A recent article in *Inquiry*, the Blue Cross Association journal, challenges Blue Cross/Blue Shield to innovation in this broad area, perhaps on a joint venture basis with some of the religious multihospital systems.[66] As another example, the insurance industry could well decide to assume primary responsibility for promoting the exciting life care or continuing care retirement community concept, which could probably profit from some additional managerial and actuarial expertise.[21a,66a]

A recent review of developments in European health care systems,[67] most of which have been experiencing the same financial problems as those of the United States, and of proposed modifications in such systems concludes that the future belongs to a public/private mix. The following refers specifically to The Netherlands but, by implication, to most of the continent:

It seems probable that the division of the population into two groups according to income level will be abolished, implying one uniform system for all people. At the same time it can be expected that market forces will be incorporated into the system. The most likely outcome will be a uniform public insurance scheme covering a minimum set of benefits, to be accompanied by regulated private insurance.

Some might say that such a formula could apply equally to the United States. If agreement could be reached on such a fundamental issue, research could then focus on the nature of the approximate mix, especially in the LTC field, and incentives relating thereto.

A major problem for both public and private insurers is the lack of adequate information as to the risk. For example, we do

---

*Over a decade ago, H. M. Somers and I suggested one such approach—a National Health Insurance model of "regulated competition" based at least partly on the Federal Employees Health Benefits Program. Under our plan, a limited number of approved public and private carriers would be permitted to compete for membership enrollment. But coverage of all Americans would be assured through a Social Security type of financing supplemented by general revenue funds. And all approved carriers would have to provide a basic package of defined benefits. (Somers, H. M. and A. R., Major issues in national health insurance, Milbank Memorial Fund Quarterly, Vol. 1: Part I, pp. 177-210, 1972. Excerpted in Somers, H. M. and A. R., Health and Health Care: Policies in Perspective, Germantown, Md.: Aspen Systems Corp., 1977, pp. 192-203.) If my LTC proposal were accepted, the basic package would include LTC as well as acute and preventive services. Thus the advantages of private enterprise could be combined with publicly assured universal coverage and an economical, balanced package of basic benefits.

not really know who makes up the LTC population. Are most LTC patients candidates for lifetime care? Or can they make do with intermittent care? Or some combination involving lifetime monitoring but intermittent services? How much formal support or care is necessary to sustain a reasonable level of informal or unpaid care? Better information on such questions would enable all potential carriers and agencies to better estimate both the risk and cost of LTC coverage.

With respect to nursing homes and home health agencies, the private sector is dominant. Here the division is between nonprofit and for-profit ownership. It appears, at least at the present time, that this is generally a healthy situation, conducive to innovation and constructive competition, provided that all conform to basic national and state standards respecting nondiscrimination in admissions and quality. See point 9 below.

5. *Public Responsibility: Federal vs. State/Local Governments?* Within the public arena, however defined, there is the recurring issue of which level or levels of government should be responsible for administration. Medicare is or was, until very recently, a strictly federal program. (Under new waiver authority, several states now have a large degree of control, at least over financial arrangements and provider payments. How far this devolution of responsibility will be carried remains to be seen.) In Medicaid, the federal role was much smaller to begin with and even that is being rapidly eroded. Medicaid could end up simply as another block grant for states to use pretty much as they see fit.

Demands for the reconsideration of federal/state relations recur frequently but rarely result in significant action. The flurry of activity, and even excitement, that followed President Reagan's call for a "New Federalism" in his 1982 State of the Union message has almost completely disappeared. The possibility of federalizing Medicaid in return for state assumption of several welfare programs attracted considerable attention. With respect to LTC, however, it turned out that federalization was not being seriously considered. Medicaid was to be split up into two or three segments with the LTC segment remaining with the states, but with even less adequate federal funding than today. Given the current fiscal plight of most states, the fate of LTC under such conditions would almost certainly be deterioration rather than improvement.[68]

The failure of the New Federalism proposal to generate any serious reforms, either in Medicaid or LTC, is unfortunate. Certainly there are no easy answers, but that should not discourage the effort to seek new approaches. The second part of my LTC proposal (see footnote to point 4, above) is one attempt to deal with this problem; S. 1244 provides a different approach. There are others. This too is an area in need of objective research.

6. *Public Programs: General Revenues vs. Special Taxes?* Almost all public programs providing LTC in the United States are supported by funds derived from general revenues. This includes Medicaid, the VA, titles III and XX of the Social Security Act, and state and local mental and chronic hospitals. The only exception is Medicare, whose relatively small contribution to LTC is financed in the same way as its acute care, that is, primarily through the Part A (Hospital Insurance) payroll tax. About 75 percent of the funds for Part B, originally raised on a 50/50 basis between the premium tax paid by beneficiaries and general revenues, now comes from the latter. Altogether at least 90 percent of the public money spent for LTC comes from general revenues.

Obviously, this contrasts sharply with the financing of acute care, where the proportions are roughly reversed. Does this dichotomy make sense? Is it a good way of "spreading the heat"? Or does it accentuate the Iron Curtain between acute care coverage, with its near-universal and quasi-insurance entitlement, and LTC, with its highly limited, welfare connotation? Or both? Assuming it makes sense to tear down, or at least modify, this Iron Curtain, as I have recommended,[59] with the Medicaid responsibility for LTC for the elderly and disabled transferred to Medicare, this would obviously involve a commingling of general and special revenues. If, at the same time, Medicare parts A and B were merged, this would provide further opportunity for redesigning the revenue structure. Considering the enormous sums involved in such a merged program, a great deal of study should be given to the most equitable and effective distribution of the burden between the different methods and levels of taxation.

7. *Primary Setting: Institutional vs. Community/Home?* The strong pro-institutional incentives in both Medicare and Medicaid and their expensive consequences have been recognized for

a number of years. Some apparently consider this the central issue in the entire LTC field.[69] Why the failure to take corrective action? Most obviously, the strength of the vested interests that have grown up around the current arrangements makes it exceedingly difficult to effect any significant transfer of entitlements or funds, especially in a period of serious financial constraints. Indeed, there is fear on the part of many policymakers that effective transfer is impossible and that any addition of now uncovered community- or home-based LTC benefits will inevitably end up, not as substitutions, but as "add-ons" to the existing benefit package. Moreover, they fear that any new benefits will, also inevitably, result in many new beneficiaries. Many LTC patients who are now making do at home or in some residential facility with family or other informal supports would then end up on a public program. According to this view, even if the per capita costs of caring for individual patients could be cut by substituting more community/home care for institutional care, the total costs would rise substantially. Therefore, don't make things worse than they now are!

The net result of these conflicting pressures—"Cut the costs of institutional care!" vs. "Don't open the possibility of more beneficiaries!"—has been the extensive but halfhearted LTC demonstration projects already noted. Limited in both beneficiaries (usually only to those who would otherwise require Medicaid nursing home admission) and costs (usually a ceiling of 60 to 95 percent of comparable nursing home costs), they were viewed, almost exclusively, as cheaper alternatives to nursing home care, rather than as desirable programs in their own right. The inconclusive results are consistent with earlier studies.[23,70,71] But, inconclusive or not, states are being pressured to move faster in this direction, strictly on the basis of economy. Although the unique New York State Long-Term Home Health Care Program, 1978–1982, was not a demonstration project, its results are relevant. According to an interim report, average expenditures for the 4,000 Medicaid home care patients were half the cost of an "equivalent level of institutional care."[25] An earlier study by Weissert reported that adult day care offered the possibility of savings of 37 to 60 percent compared to the cost of nursing home care on a period-of-care basis.[72]

There is a danger that the pendulum will now swing in the opposite direction, that we may repeat the earlier indiscriminate deinstitutionalization of the mentally ill, again with predictable results. Abuse and neglect are not limited to the institutional setting.[72a] Some experts on aging are already warning of this. Dr. Sidney Katz, Director of the Gerontology Center at Brown University, has pointed out that "changing social demographics will force national policy away from the philosophy of reinforcing dependence upon family and friends for help, to greater support of the role of institutions in care for the elderly."[73]

Despite the idealistic motivation of many sponsors of community- and home-based projects, there is danger that this whole development will further exacerbate the acute care vs. LTC dichotomy to the further detriment of LTC. What is badly needed, at this juncture, is recognition of the facts that both institutional and noninstitutional modalities are needed and appropriate in given situations, depending partly on the level and duration of care needed, partly on the availability of family and other informal supports; that neither patients nor their care-givers should be locked into any one modality; and that some way must be found—through objective functional assessment, case management, patient cost-sharing, appropriate reimbursement policies, tax incentives for family care, respite services, family education, etc.—to facilitate flexible access to the broad range of services that will make possible the most cost-effective, as well as health-effective, use of all our LTC resources, including long-term hospitals. Clearly, research in this area is needed, one promising possibility being the cross-cutting life care retirement community.[21,21a,74,75]

8. *Organization of Patient Care: Primary Physician vs. Case Manager.* LTC generally involves a much greater "management" function than acute care. First, the patient is likely to be older, poorer, with fewer family supports, little or no health insurance and, of course, sick or disabled for a much longer period of time. Second, the length of time over which care has to be sustained usually involves changing physical, mental, economic, and familial conditions. Third, the frequent combination of physical/mental and social/economic dependence often calls for a finely tuned interdisciplinary approach which can rarely be achieved without an individual organizer or manager.

Recently a new twist has been added—the "gatekeeper" concept. The gatekeeper is a generalist who has overall responsibility for the patient and without whose permission or referral, specialist care will not be paid by a third party.[76] The concept is by no means limited to LTC. In fact it is currently more common in HMOs, "primary care networks," and other forms of "alternative" care for younger populations. However, it is related to the case manager function and is an intrinsic part of the experimental S/HMO model.

Assuming that some form of the case manager becomes increasingly common in LTC, for the reasons noted above, the important question then arises: who shall it be? At least three options are theoretically possible: (1) We could return to the traditional general practitioner or family doctor, require all LTC patients to register with one, and make him or her responsible for all referrals, medical and social. (2) We could set up a separate system for LTC patients, using a nurse practitioner, social worker, or other nonphysician as case manager, with full responsibility for referrals. (3) We could devise some compromise between 1 and 2, assigning final professional, legal, and moral responsibility to a physician but encouraging delegation of nonmedical referrals to an associated nonphysician. The financing incentives and implications of the different alternatives are important. Here again I have tried to develop at least the outline of some such approach,[59] but the whole issue needs much more study.

9. *Cost Controls: Competition vs. Regulation?* It is surely unnecessary to document further the need for cost controls in any viable LTC program. Nor is it necessary to review the multifaceted debate over competition vs. regulation that has enlivened the health care scene during the past few years. It is significant, however, that the "pro-competition" advocates rarely point to LTC as an area particularly well suited to the free market and price competition. On the contrary, the absence of private insurance from the LTC field emphasizes the generally poor fit between the LTC market and pure competition.

Two exceptions have been noted: the proprietary nursing home and the new field of proprietary home care agencies. Although the majority of homes are operated for profit (Table 2a), they now operate within a highly regulated environment which proved necessary as a result of extensive abuses in the early days of proprietary expansion. Efforts on the part of the Reagan Administration to reduce federal nursing home regulations, especially with respect to inspection and accreditation, have thus far been resisted by Congress and consumer groups. A new approach, involving creation of an independent commission to reexamine the whole question of nursing home quality standards and controls, is far more promising.

The for-profit home health agencies are less regulated, a cause for concern. Although there have never been the abuses or even allegations of abuses such as characterized the nursing home industry 15 years ago, the potential for serious abuse is even greater. It is hard to imagine a more vulnerable individual than an 85-year-old widow, aphasic and paralyzed from stroke, living alone in a rural area or high-crime inner city. It is inconceivable that any third party, public or private, would ever sanction, through reimbursement or otherwise, the entry of alimentation technicians, "homemakers," "home health aides," "chore workers" or paraprofessionals of any other category into such a home except on a regulated basis.

Neither regulation nor competition alone can solve all the problems of this complex industry.[4,11,77] What is needed is a flexible mixture, and this is another area for study.

10. *Patient Cost-Sharing: Deterrence vs. Assistance?* Recent confirmation of the commonsense notion that deductibles and co-insurance reduce the use of health services by average healthy individuals under age 65[78] is hardly a breathtaking discovery. The problem of cost-sharing by the elderly, especially for LTC, is as complex as it is important. The usual argument against cost-sharing, the danger of underutilization, has to be carefully balanced against a potential advantage: the possibility of providing coverage to hitherto excluded individuals or of improving existing benefits. For example, if reasonable cost-sharing could make possible universal Medicare coverage of a reasonable amount of LTC services, as opposed to the current general exclusion, it would obviously be a positive step for most of the elderly. To determine the viability and the terms of such a trade-off would require study of a number of issues including:

- effect of various cost-sharing formulas on the price of specific LTC services,
- effect on the use of such services,
- effect on patient health,
- potential for expanding coverage of such services,
- potential for covering new benefits, and

- administrative feasibility and effect on costs of administration.

Two related approaches deserve consideration: (1) voluntary supplementation of LTC costs paid by a public program, now generally illegal under Medicaid, and (2) tax incentives to encourage and help families to take care of patients at home.[4] H.R. 3036, authorizing the latter, was introduced by Congressman Rinaldo.

11. *Payment of Institutional Providers: Prospective vs. Retrospective Rates?* The absurdity of the "reasonable costs" approach to hospital reimbursement and its enormous inflationary impact on the costs of health insurance have been recognized by health care authorities for years. Nevertheless it took nearly 18 years and the prospect of bankruptcy for the Medicare Hospital Insurance Trust Fund before Congress became willing to undertake serious corrective action. Now with the shift to diagnosis-related groups (DRGs) incentives are being totally reversed and concern shifts from the likelihood of overutilization to the possibility of underutilization.[79] Hopefully, the gradual phasing in of the new program and provision for complicated cases and other exceptional circumstances ("outliers") will permit this experiment to be more successful than the previous one.

At the moment, chronic hospitals and other LTC institutions are exempt from the DRG experiment. This was certainly wise. The feasibility of applying this methodology to LTC has yet to be demonstrated and at first glance seems unlikely. The very thought of using the payment mechanism to try to speed up patient discharge from an LTC facility or program appears a contradiction in terms. If a speedy cure had been possible, the patient would not be on LTC at all. Moreover, many LTC patients defy being "pigeonholed" into a single diagnostic category. Multiple pathologies are the rule rather than the exception with the very old. Then, too, in the LTC field, unlike acute care, underutilization is already a widespread problem.[11]

This is not to imply that retroactive cost-based reimbursement is any more appropriate for LTC than for acute care. But the alternative is not necessarily per case reimbursement. Payment based on fixed prices or charges per diem, per week, or per month, is also an alternative. The per-case system not only calls for fixed prices but also changes the unit or "product" being priced, from time unit—a day—to a cause of disability. Obviously this is a good way to get at alleged overutilization, but since this is not generally the problem in LTC, some other more relevant alternative will probably have to be sought. Among those suggested: a point system, perhaps based on an activities of daily living index, which would reward admission to heavy-care patients (already being tried out in a few states), or an outcome-oriented system with payment based on whether the patient does better or worse than predicted by some neutral analyst.[4,17,80] The congressional proposal noted above to establish an independent commission to review federal nursing home standards could also provide a highly appropriate opportunity for simultaneous study of reimbursement.[81]

12. *Payment of Practitioners: Fee-for-Service vs. Capitation/ Salary?* Current interest in HMOs, preferred provider organizations, and related "alternative delivery systems" stems from much the same concern as the DRG movement. It is widely alleged that fee-for-service payment prompts overutilization of physician and other professional services while capitation or salary encourages more restrained and therefore more appropriate and less expensive use of services. As already noted in connection with institutional payment, testing this hypothesis is exceptionally difficult in the LTC field. It will be equally so for practitioners. Good geriatric doctors and nurses are very scare, regardless of how, or how much, they are paid.

Hopefully, the S/HMO experiment will shed some light on this issue, although it is not clear how much use will be made of physicians in these projects. In any case, the crucial case manager function, whether performed by a physician or nonphysician, obviously has to be paid on a salary or capitation basis. If the entire array of home care personnel, including visiting nurses and therapists, could be maintained on a salaried basis, it would probably be much less expensive than fee for service. But is this possible or equitable, if most physicians continue to work on a fee-for-service basis? These are not easily researchable issues, but they are crucial to the viable financing, i.e., the success, of any large-scale LTC program.

Perhaps even more urgent, in my view, are the issues of (1) selective "assignment," which permits physicians to pick and choose among their patients as to whom they will bill above Medicare rates; and (2) the strong protechnology bias in existing Medicare and most private health insurance fee structures.

This is indeed a formidable agenda—but so is the challenge. In the words of one physician, Dr. Nicholas Rango:[11]

Unless the needs of present and future cohorts of the dependent elderly are soon addressed, a policy crisis of awesome economic, political, and moral dimensions will occur. It is past time for society to decide how it will provide for its elderly members who are delivered by modern medicine into an unprecedented and uncertain state of survivorship with extreme impairment.

REFERENCES

1. Somers, A. R., Fabian D. R. (eds.). The Geriatric Imperative: An Introduction to Gerontology and Clinical Geriatrics. New York: Appleton-Century-Crofts, 1981.

2. Liu, K., Palesch, Y. The nursing home population: Different perspectives and implications for policy. Health Care Financing Review 3 (December):15-23.

3. Department of Health, Education and Welfare, National Center for Health Statistics. The National Nursing Home Survey: 1977 Summary for the United States. DHEW Publ. No. (PHS) 79-1794, Hyattsville, Md.: 1979.

4. Department of Health and Human Services, Office of the Inspector General. Long-Term Care. Service Delivery Assessment. Report to the Secretary, 1981 (unpublished), 2 vols.

5. Somers, A. R. Marital status, health and the use of health services: An old relationship revisited. Journal of the American Medical Association 241:1818-22, 1979.

6. Freeland, M., Schendler, C. E. National health expenditure growth in the 1980s: An aging population, new technologies, and increasing competition. Health Care Financing Review 4 (March):18, 1983.

7. Gibson, R. M., Waldo, D. R. National health expenditures, 1980. Health Care Financing Review 3 (March): 1-54, 1981.

8. Fisher, C. R. Differences by age group in health care spending. Health Care Financing Review 1 (Spring):65-90, 1980. (Data for 1978, the latest available.)

9. Kovar, M. G. (National Center for Health Statistics): The U.S. elderly people and their medical care. Background paper for Commonwealth Forum, Improving the Health of the Homebound Elderly, 1983 (unpublished).

10. Vladeck, B. C. Nursing homes. In Mechanic, D. (ed), Handbook of Health, Health Care, and the Health Professions. Riverside, NJ: 1983, pp. 352-364.

11. Rango, N. Nursing home care in the U.S.: Prevailing conditions and policy implications. New England Journal of Medicine 307:883-889, 1982.

12. Garibaldi, R. A., Brodine S., Matsuniga S. Infections among patients in nursing homes. New England Journal of Medicine 305:731-35, 1981.

12a. U.S. General Accounting Office. Preliminary Findings on Patient Characteristics and State Medicaid Expenditures for Nursing Home Care. Report to the Chairman, Subcommittee on Health and the Environment of the Committee on Energy and Commerce, Washington, D.C., GAO/IPE-82-4, 1982.

13. Department of Health and Human Services, Office of the Inspector General. Service Delivery Assessment. Restricted Patient Admittance to Nursing Homes: An Assessment of Hospital Backup. Report to the Secretary, 1980 (unpublished).

14. Van Nostrand, J. F. (National Center for Health Statistics). Personal communication, June 29, 1983.

15. Eidus, R. The physician and the nursing home patient. In Somers, A. R., and Fabian, D. R. (eds.). The Geriatric Imperative: An Introduction to Gerontology and Clinical Geriatrics. New York: Appleton-Century-Crofts, 1981.

16. Butler, R. B. The teaching nursing home. Journal of the American Medical Association 245:1435-37, 1981.

17. Kane, R. L., et al. Predicting the outcome of the nursing home patients. The Gerontologist 23:200-206, 1983.

18. McCaffree, K. M. Profits, Growth, and Reimbursement Systems in the Nursing Home Industry. Baltimore, Md.: Health Care Financing Administration Publication No. 03097, 1981.

19. Department of Health and Human Services, Health Care Financing Administration. Long-Term Care: Background and Future Directions. Washington, D.C.: 1981.

20. Vladeck, B. C. Understanding long-term care. New England Journal of Medicine, 307:889-890, 1982.

21. Human Services Research Inc. 1982 Reference Directory of Continuing Care Retirement Communities. Philadelphia, 1982.

21a. Winklevoss, H. E., Powell, A. V. Continuing Care Retirement Communities: An Empirical, Financial, and Legal Analysis. Homewood, Ill.: Richard D. Irwin, 1983.

22. McLaughlin, S. (National Association for Home Care.) Washington, D.C. Personal communication, June 30, 1983.

23. Spiegel, A. D. Home Health Care: Home Birthing to Hospice Care. Owings Mills, Md.: National Health Publishing, 1983.

24. Cherkasky, M. The Montefiore Hospital Home Care Program. American Journal of Public Health 39 (February):29-20, 1949.

25. Brickner, P. W. Ten Years of Long-Term Home Health Care, January 1973–December 1982. New York: St. Vincent's Hospital and Medical Center, 1983.

26. Iglehart, J. K. Funding the End-Stage Renal Disease Program. New England Journal of Medicine 306:492-496, 1982.

27. Kleinfield, N. R. The home health care boom: High tech spurs field. New York Times, June 30, 1983.

28. Home Health Line, Vol. VI, February 26, 1982, p. 2. Data from Health Care Financing Administration.

29. Muse, D. N., Sawyer, D. Medicare and Medicaid Data Book, 1981. Baltimore, Md.: Health Care Financing Administration Publication No. 03128, 1982.

30. Health Care Financing Administration. Medicare and Medicaid Data Book, 1983.

31. Anderson, A. (Health Research and Educational Trust, Princeton, N.J.) Personal communication, July 5, 1983.

32. Department of Health and Human Services, National Center for Health Statistics. Health U.S.—1982. DHHS Publ. No. (PHS)83-1232, Hyattsville, Md.: 1983, pp. 80-81.

33. Loeser, W. D, Dickstein, E. S., Schiavone, L. D. Medicare coverage in nursing homes—a broken promise. New England Journal of Medicine 304:353-354, 1981.

34. Pear, R. Medicare predicts insolvency of fund by 1990. New York Times, June 24, 1983. (About Federal Hospital Insurance Trust Fund, Trustees Report, 1983.)

35. U.S. Senate. Special Committee on Aging. Action on Aging Legislation in 97th Congress. 98th Cong. First Sess. Senate Print 98-14. Washington, D.C.: Government Printing Office, 1983.

36. U.S. Senate. Special Committee on Aging. Proposed Fiscal Year 1984 Budget: What It Means for Older Americans. 98th Cong. First Sess. Senate Print 98-19. Washington, D.C.: Government Printing Office, 1983.

37. Bureau of the Census. Preliminary Estimates of the Population of the U.S., by Age, Sex, and Race: 1970-1981. Current Population Reports. Washington, D.C.: Ser. P-25, No. 917, July 1982.

38. Clinkscale, R., et al. Analysis of State Medicaid Program Characteristics 1982. Rockville, Md.: Health Care Financing Administration, Office of Research and Demonstrations and LaJolla Management Corp. (unpublished).

39. Mitchell, J. B., Cromwell, J. Medicaid mills: fact or fiction? Health Care Financing Review 2 (Summer):37-49, 1980.

40. Congressional Budget Office. Long-Term Care for the Elderly and Disabled. Washington, D.C., 1977, p. 24.

41. Vladeck, B. C. Unloving Care: The Nursing Home Tragedy. New York: Basic Books, 1980, p. 24.

42. Altman, D. Health care for the poor. Annals of the American Academy of Political and Social Science, July 1983.

42a. Schram, S. F. Social services for older people. In Neugarten, B.L. (ed.), Age or Need? Public Policies for Older People. Beverly Hills, Calif: Sage Publications, 1982, pp. 221-246.

43. Hickman, D. (National Association of Area Agencies on Aging, Washington, D.C.) Personal communication, July 5, 1983.

44. Ayres, B. D. VA may face crisis as veterans turn 65 and seek free care. New York Times, February 26, 1983.

45. Day, B. Aging vets challenge VA future. VA Vanguard, Washington, D.C.: 29 (May):6-9, 1983.

46. Veterans Administration. Caring for the Older Veteran: Report of the Special Medical Advisory Group Task Force on the VA Geriatric Plan. Washington, D.C., 1983.

47. U.S. General Accounting Office. The Elderly Should Benefit From Expanded Home Health Care but Increasing These Services Will Not Insure Cost Reductions. Washington, D.C., GAO/IPE-83-1, 1982.

48. Health Care Financing Administration. Briefing Materials: National Long-Term Care Channeling Demonstration. Assistant Secretary for Planning and Evaluation, Washington, D.C., (January 11) 1983.

49. Diamond, L. M., et al. Eldercare for the 1980s: Health and social service in one prepaid health maintenance system. The Gerontologist 23:148-154, 1983.

50. Somers, A. R., Kleinman L., Clark, W. D. Preventive health services for the elderly: The Rutgers Medical School project. Inquiry 19:190-198, 1982.

51. Greenlick, M. R., et al. Kaiser-Permanente's Medicare Plus Project: A successful Medicare prospective payment demonstration. Health Care Financing Review 4 (Summer):85-97, 1983.

52. Clines, F. X. Reagan asks doctors to support freeze in their Medicare returns. New York Times, June 24, 1983.

53. Somers, A. R. Rethinking Medicare to Meet Future Needs. Washington, D.C.: Government Research Corp., 1982.

54. Vladeck, B.C. Understanding long-term care. New England Journal of Medicine 307:889-890, 1982.

55. United Kingdom Department of Health and Social Security. Health Care and Its Costs. London: HMSO, 1983. (Reported in British Information Services, Survey of Current Affairs 13, May 5, 1983, pp. 175-176.)

56. Williams, M. E., Hadler, H. M. The illness is the focus of geriatric medicine. New England Journal of Medicine 308:1357-1359, 1983.

57. Kennie, D. C. Good health care for the aged. Journal of the American Medical Association 249:770-773, 1983.

58. Friggens, P. Easing the problems of aging: An interview with Dr. R. N. Butler. Exxon USA Magazine (Houston) First Quarter 1983:12-15.

59. Somers, A. R. Long-term care for the elderly and disabled: A new health priority. New England Journal of Medicine 307:221-226, 1982.

60. Ruchlin, H. S., et al. Management and funding of long-term care services: A new approach to a chronic problem. New England Journal of Medicine 306:101-106, 1982.

61. Murphy, J. F. The role of the insurance industry in long-term care. In Home Health Agency Assembly of New Jersey (et al.), Proceedings of an Invitational Conference: Broadening Access to Long-Term Care. Piscataway, N.J., 1982, pp. 27-30.

62. Slattery, R. M. Private insurance. In Home Health Agency Assembly of New Jersey (et al.), Proceedings of an Invitational Conference: Broadening Access to Long-Term Care. Piscataway, N.J., 1982, pp. 63-70.

63. Meiners, M. R. The case of long-term care insurance. Health Affairs 2 (Summer):55-79, 1983.

64. Minard, D. E. A role for insurance. In Home Health Agency Assembly of New Jersey (et al.), Proceedings of an Invitational Conference: Broadening Access to Long-Term Care. Piscataway, N.J., 1982, pp. 71-75.

65. Firman, J. Reforming community care for the elderly and disabled. Health Affairs 2 (Spring):66-82, 1983.

66. Griffith, J. R. The role of Blue Cross and Blue Shield in the future U.S. health care system. Inquiry 20 (Spring):12-19, 1983.

66a. Rudvitsky, H., Konrad, W. Trouble in the elysian fields. Forbes, August 29, 1983.

67. Rutten, F.F. H. Health care policy today: Making way for the libertarians? Effective Health Care (Amsterdam) 1 (June):35-43, 1983.

68. Somers, A. R. Long-term care for the elderly and disabled: An urgent challenge to the "New Federalism." Paper presented to Project Hope, Conference on the New Federalism and Long-Term Care for the Elderly, Millwood, Va., December 10, 1982.

69. Laurence, D. B., Gaus, C. R. Long-term care: Financing and policy issues. In Mechanic, D. (ed.), Handbook of Health, Health Care, and the Health Professions. New York: Free Press, 1983, pp. 365-378.

70. Hammon, J. Home health care cost effectiveness: An overview of the literature. Public Health Reports 94:205-211, 1979.

71. Dunlop, B. D. Expanded home-based care for the impaired elderly: Solution or pipe dream? American Journal of Public Health 70:514-519, 1980.

72. Weissert, W. G. Costs of adult day care: A comparison to nursing homes. Inquiry XV (March):10-19, 1978.

72a. Hickey, T., Douglass, R. L. Mistreatment of the elderly in the domestic setting—an exploratory study. American Journal of Public Health 71:500-507, 1981.

73. Stuart, R. "Old-old" grow in number and impact. New York Times, June 20, 1983.

74. Lanahan, M. B. Life care retirement communities. Pride Institute. Journal of Long-Term Care Home Health Care 2 (Spring):41-42, 1983.

75. Fillenbaum, G. G. Portrait of a life-care community: An alternate living arrangement for the elderly. Durham, N.C.: Duke University Center for the Study of Aging and Human Development, Center Reports on Advances in Research 5, 1981.

76. Somers, A. R. And who shall be the gatekeeper? Inquiry 20 (Winter) 1983.

77. Spiegel, A. D, et al. Issues and opportunities in the regulation of home health care. Health Policy and Education (Amsterdam) 1:237-253, 1980.

78. Newhouse, J. P., et al. Some interim results from a controlled trial of cost-sharing in health insurance. New England Journal of Medicine 305:1501-1507, 1981.

79. Garber, A. M., Fuchs, V. R., Silverman, J. F. Case Mix, Costs, and Outcomes: Differences between Faculty and Community Services in a University Hospital. Stanford, Calif.: National Bureau of Economic Research Working Paper No. 1159, 1983.

80. Weissert, W. G., et al. Encouraging appropriate care for the chronically ill: Design of the National Center for Health Services research experiment in nursing home incentive payments. Paper presented to Meeting of the American Public Health Association, Detroit 1980.

81. Edwards, C. (American Association of Homes for the Aged.) Personal communication, July 18, 1983.

Index

A

Abusive behavior, 161–162
Acetylcholine, 115, 142
Active life expectancy, 10, 57–72
  concept development, 58–64
  policy implications, 64–69
  statistics, 57–58
Activities of Daily Living Index,
  10, 57, 60–64
Adrenocorticotropic hormone
  (ACTH), 115, 120
Ageism, 118
Aging process
  as disease, 73
  See also Demography
Aluminum, 144, 146
Alzheimer, Alois, 141
Alzheimer's disease, 13, 109, 138,
  139
  incidence, 13, 22, 37, 40
  mechanism, 141–145
  related issues, 146–148
  risk factors, 145–146
  support groups, 168
  symptoms, 140–141
Amitriptyline (Elavil), 122
Amphetamines, 122

Antianxiety drugs, 109
Anticholinergic effects, 122, 123
Antidepressant drugs, 112, 121–
  124
Arterial aging. *See*
  Cardiovascular aging
Arteriosclerosis, 34, 35
Atherosclerosis, 11, 34, 75–80,
  100–101
Atypical depression, 109
Autonomous depression, 108
Aventyl, 122

B

Barbiturates, 109
Beck, John C., 10, 57–72
Benzodiazepines, 112
Bereavement, 107, 118
Beta-adrenergic response, 95–101
Beta-blocking drugs, 109
Blazer, Dan, 14, 105–128
Blood pressure
  age/increase relationship, 86–
    89, 101
  hypertension, 34
Blue Cross/Blue Shield, 220

Brain tumors, 139
Branch, Laurence G., 10, 57–72

C

Cancer, 33, 35
Cardiac hypertrophy, 86, 88, 101
Cardiac output. *See*
    Cardiovascular aging
Cardiovascular aging, 22, 73–104
    atherosclerosis, 75–80
    and dementia, 138
    exercise tolerance decline, 89–
        100
    life style variables, 80–81
    mechanism, 82–83
    resting cardiac output, age
        effects on, 83–89
    summary, 11–12, 73–75, 100–
        102
Cardiovascular diseases, 33–35
Case managers, 224–225, 228
Catecholamine secretion, 95–96,
    101, 115, 121
Cerebral arteriosclerosis, 144
Cerebral vascular disease, 33–35
Chlordiazepoxide (Librium), 112
Cholecystokinin, 143
Choline, 144
Choline acetyltransferase, 142–
    143, 146
Cholinergic system, 142–145
Chromosome 21, 146
Chronic organic brain syndrome,
    12–13, 136
Circadian rhythms, 124
Cognition. *See* Dementia
Community programs
    demonstration projects, 211–
        214, 223
    expenditures, 185, 194
    federal funding, 208–209
    independent community care
        program, 214–215
    institutionalization versus,
        222–224

long-term care industry, 194–
    198
support groups, 165–168, 174
Community Services Block Grant
    program, 208
Cortisol, 109, 115
Costs and expenditures
    Alzheimer's disease, 146–147
    community-based care, 185, **194**
    cost controls, 225–226
    dementia diagnostic tests, 139–
        140
    financial incentives for
        informal support systems,
        172, 227
    informal long-term care, 157–
        158, 172
    long-term care industry, 185
    long-term hospitals, 185, 198–
        200
    nursing homes, 64–65, 185,
        187, 193
    overview, 42–44
    patient cost-sharing, 226–227
    payment methods, 227–229
    See also Financing programs;
        Medicaid and Medicare

D

Dalmane, 109
Dementia, 12–14, 129–140
    aging/cognition relationship,
        12, 22, 129–135
    causes of, 138–139
    definition of, 135–136
    dexamethasone suppression
        test, 120
    diagnostic tests, costs of, 139–
        140
    incidence, 13, 136–138
    pharmacological therapy, 122
    See also Alzheimer's disease
Demography, 1–6, 28–47
    active life expectancy, 58–59,
        67–68

care-givers, by sex, 158, 159,
170
changes within aged
population, 21, 29–31
income and expenditures, 8–9,
45–47
life expectancy, 10
marriage statistics, 154
medical care costs, 42–44
morbidity statistics, 3–4, 9–11,
15, 35–38
mortality statistics, 31–35, 59
use of services, 39–42
Demoralization, 107
Depressive illness, 14, 22, 105–
128
biological and psychological
origins, 113–119
burden of, 110–113
characteristics of, 106–110
diagnostic tests, 119–121
incidence, 37, 110–113
origins, 113–119
treatment, 112–113, 121–125
Desyrel, 123
Dexamethasone suppression, 115,
120
Diagnostic tests
for dementia, 139–140
for depressive illness, 119–121
Diazepam (Valium), 109, 112
Disability, 2, 6
Down's syndrome, 145–146
Doxepin (Sinequan), 122
Drugs
misuse or intoxication, 14, 109,
112, 122
nursing home use, 17

E

Echocardiography, 88
Elavil, 122
Electrocardiography, 77, 78
Electroconvulsive therapy, 123
Endocrine disturbances, 115

Episodic short-term memory,
134–135
Exercise
sports records, 133–134
tolerance, 11–12, 80–81, 89–
101

F

Financing programs, 24, 200–215
community demonstration
projects, 211–214
independent community care
program, 214–215
Older Americans Act, 208–209
private health insurance, 43,
46, 65, 201, 203–204, 219–
221
public/private expenditures,
200–201
public/private responsibilities,
219–222
revenue sources, 222
Social Security Act, Title XX,
207–208
Veterans Administration, 64,
209–211
See also Medicaid and Medicare
Fiscal responsibility, 171–172
Flurazepam (Dalmane), 109
Frail elderly, 3, 153–181
Friendships, 155

G

Gamma-aminobutyric acid
neurons, 143
Genetic predisposition
to Alzheimer's disease, 144, 145
to depressive illness, 116
Greer, David S., 10, 57–72

H

Hartford Foundation-Rutgers
Medical School Geriatrics
Demonstration Project, 213

Health care. *See* Community
  programs; Informal support
  systems; Long-term care
Health care costs. *See* Costs and
  expenditures; Financing
  programs; Medicaid and
  Medicare
Health insurance, 43
  and long-term care, 65, 201,
    203–204, 219–221
  use and coverage, 46
  See also Medicaid and Medicare
Health maintenance
  organizations, 48
Heart disease, 33–35
Home care
  home health services, 40–41,
    47, 195–198, 202–203, 214–
    215, 225, 226
  See also Informal support
    systems
Hospice care, 48, 52, 194
Hospitalization
  for depressive illness, 124
  long-term hospitals, 185, 198–
    200, 222
  use statistics, 39–40
  Veterans Administration
    programs, 209–210
Hydergine, 122
Hydrocephalus, 139
Hypertension, 34
Hypochondriasis, 109

I

Immunologic changes, 146
Income statistics, 8–9, 45–47
Inderal, 109
Indoleamines, 115
Informal support systems, 153–
  181
  costs of family care, 157–158,
    172
  effects of care-giving on, 162–
    165

existing social networks, 154–
  157
future capabilities, 168–171
institutionalization versus,
  222–224
long-term care given by, 157–
  162
policy considerations, 171–175
summary, 8, 16, 153, 175–176
unmet needs, 165–168
Insurance. *See* Health insurance;
  Medicaid and Medicare
Intelligence. *See* Dementia
International Atherosclerosis
  Project, 75
Ischemic heart disease, 77–78

K

Kaiser-Permanente Medical Care
  Program, 213
Katz, Sidney, 10, 20, 57–72
Katzman, Robert, 12–14, 129–
  152
Kerr-Mills Medical Assistance for
  the Aged, 204

L

Lakatta, Edward G., 11–12, 73–
  104
Learned helplessness, 14, 117
Lecithin, 144
Librium, 112
Life expectancy, 10. *See also*
  Active life expectancy
Life style variables
  and cardiovascular functioning,
    11, 74, 80–81
  social networks, 154–157
Loneliness, 155
Long-term care (LTC), 2
  active life expectancy,
    implications, 63, 65–67
  community programs, 194–198
  conclusions and
    recommendations, 20–25

cost controls, 225–226
definition and focus of, 6, 182–185, 216–217
expenditures, 185
financing programs, 200–215
funding concerns, 219–222
hospitals, 198–200
institutionalization versus home setting, 222–224
issues identified, 3–9, 14–20, 49–53, 215–229
mainstream versus separate system, 218–219
Medicaid/Medicare eligibility, 217–218
patient cost-sharing, 226–227
payment methods, 227–229
physician versus case manager, 224–225

M

Malignant neoplasms, 33
Marriage statistics, 154
Medicaid and Medicare, 4, 8, 16, 18, 23, 28, 52, 53, 65, 184, 215
Alzheimer's disease, 147
coverage and expenditures data, 42–44, 46, 49, 200–207
demonstration projects, 212
and family care-giving, 156, 172, 173
federal and state responsibilities, 221–222
home health services, 41, 47, 197–198, 202–203
independent community care project, 214–215
nursing homes, 18, 40, 46–47, 64, 187, 191–193, 202, 204–205
program changes, 47–49, 217–218
revenue sources, 222

service use changes induced by, 39, 41–42
Medical Costs. *See* Costs and expenditures; Financing programs; Medicaid and Medicare
Medical Retirement Account, 219
Memory, 134–135. *See also* Dementia
Methylphenidate (Ritalin), 122
Mongolism, 145–146
Monoamine oxidase inhibitors, 109
Morbidity statistics, 3–4, 9–11, 15, 35–38
Mortality statistics, 31–35, 59
Motivation, 118
Multi-infarct dementia, 13, 138

N

Netherlands, 220
Neuroendocrine system, 115
Neurotransmitter abnormalities, 113, 115, 142–144
New York State Long-Term Home Health Care Program, 213, 223
Noradrenalin, 143
Norepinephrine, 115, 122
Nortriptyline (Aventyl, Pamelor), 122
Nursing Home Without Walls programs, 213
Nursing homes, 16–20, 168, 172, 185–193, 225–226
classification of, 191
drug use, 17
expenditures, 64–65, 185, 187, 193
home and bed statistics, 187–191
length-of-stay data, 191–192
Medicaid/Medicare coverage, 18, 40, 46–47, 64, 187, 191–193, 202, 204–205

monthly charges, 193
staffing, 192
use statistics, 37, 40, 47, 185–187

O

Older Americans Act of 1965, 208–209
Oregon, 213

P

Packwood-Bradley-Heinz bill, 214–215, 219
Pamelor, 122
Parkinson's disease, 109, 131–132
Payment. *See* Costs and expenditures; Financing programs; Medicaid and Medicare
Pharmacological therapy, 109, 112, 121–124
Phenothiazines, 112
Physical activity. *See* Exercise
Physician visits, 39, 224–225
Physostigmine, 144
Pituitary functioning, 115, 120
Precursor therapy, 144–145
Propranolol (Inderal), 109
Protyreline, 120
Pseudodementia, 37, 109
Psychological etiology of depressive illness, 107–108, 116–119
Psychotherapy, 112, 123–124

R

Rabin, David L., 8, 17, 18, 28–56
Radioactive tracer method, 78
Radionuclide imaging, 77
Research issues, 67–68
Reserpine, 109
Retirement community, 194
Ritalin, 122
Robert Wood Johnson Foundation, 213, 219

S

Scopolamine, 143
Sedative-hypnotic drugs, 109
Senile dementia. *See* Alzheimer's disease; Dementia
Senior Citizens Independent Community Care Act, 214–215
Serotonin, 115, 122
Service use, 39–42
Silverstone, Barbara, 8, 16, 153–181
Sinequan, 122
Sleep problems, 109, 116, 120–121, 125
Smoking, 34–35
Social Health Maintenance Organization, 213, 219
Social Security, 45, 156, 171
Social Security Act, 207–208, 214, 222
Social support. *See* Informal support systems
Somatostatin, 143, 144
Somers, Anne R., 8, 15–18, 20, 182–233
Spector, William D., 10, 57–72
Sports records, 133–134
Stimulants, 122
Stress
    cardiovascular response to, 89–100
    emotional adjustment to, 107, 118–119
    See also Exercise
Strokes, 34
Subdural hematomas, 139
Substantia nigra, 131–132
Suicide, 14, 111–112
Supplemental Security Income, 173

T

Tax credits, 172, 227
Thallium scanning, 78

Thiamine deficiency, 138
Thyroid functioning, 115, 120,
    122, 138
Thyroid stimulating hormone
    (TSH), 115, 120
Thyrotropin releasing hormone
    (TRH), 115, 120
Timed tests, 133
Trazodone (Desyrel), 123
Tricyclic antidepressants, 121–
    122
Triiodothyronine, 122
Trisomy 21, 145–146

U

United Kingdom, 215

V

Valium, 109, 112
Vascular aging. *See*
    Cardiovascular aging
Vasoactive intestinal peptide, 143
Veterans Administration
    programs, 64, 209–211, 222
Viruses, 144, 146
Vitamin deficiencies, 138